Comparing Psychoanalytic Psychotherapies

- DEVELOPMENTAL, SELF, AND OBJECT RELATIONS
- SELF PSYCHOLOGY
- SHORT-TERM DYNAMIC

T0383592

Comparing Psychoanalytic Psychotherapies

- DEVELOPMENTAL, SELF, AND OBJECT RELATIONS
- SELF PSYCHOLOGY
- SHORT-TERM DYNAMIC

James F. Masterson, M.D.
Marian Tolpin, M.D.
Peter E. Sifneos, M.D.

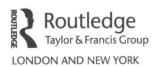
Routledge
Taylor & Francis Group

LONDON AND NEW YORK

First published 1991 by BRUNNER/MAZEL, INC.

Published 2014 by Routledge
2 Park Square, Milton Park, Abingdon, Oxfordshire OX14 4RN
711 Third Avenue, New York, NY 10017

First issued in paperback 2014

Routledge is an imprint of the Taylor & Francis Group, an informa business

Library of Congress Cataloging-in-Publication Data
Comparing psychoanalytic psychotherapies : developmental, self, and
object relations : self psychology, short-term dynamic / James F.
Masterson, Marian Tolpin, Peter E. Sifneos [panelists].
    p.   cm.
Based on two workshops held Feb. 23–24, 1990 in New York and
Mar. 9–10, 1990 San Francisco, Calif.
Includes bibliographical references.
    ISBN 978-0-87630-640-6 (hbk)
    ISBN 978-1-13800-489-4 (pbk)

    1. Borderline personality disorder—Case studies—Congresses.
2. Narcissism—Case studies—Congresses.   3. Self psychology—
Congresses.   4. Object relations (Psychoanalysis)—Congresses.
5. Brief psychotherapy—Congresses.   6. Psychodynamic psychotherapy—
Congresses.   I. Masterson, James F.   II. Tolpin, Marian.
III. Sifneos, Peter E. (Peter Emanuel)
    [DNLM: 1. Borderline Personality Disorders—congresses.
2. Narcissism—congresses.   3. Object Attachment—congresses.
4. Personality Development—congresses.   5. Psychoanalytic Therapy—
congresses.   6. Psychotherapy, Brief—congresses. WM460.6 C737
1990]
RC569.5.B67C66   1991
616.85′852—dc20
DNLM/DLC
for Library of Congress   91-8288
                                                            CIP

Contents

PART II. WORKSHOPS

PART III. OVERVIEW

Introduction

Theoretical approaches to the psychotherapy of patients with Borderline and Narcissistic Personality Disorders have grown and matured over the last 30 years. An ever increasing need has arisen for a dialogue between contrasting approaches to better define their similarities and differences.

This book reports a conference that featured a clinical dialogue between three pioneering psychotherapists to compare and contrast the approaches to psychotherapy of the Borderline and Narcissistic Personality Disorders of the developmental, self, and object relations theory and self psychology theory. In addition, it contrasts these two approaches with the short-term dynamic approach to the neuroses. It addresses two sets of questions:

How do these two theories compare with regard to:
1. Their concept of the central psychopathology of these two disorders?
2. Their view of differential diagnosis?
3. The types of therapeutic techniques they use?
4. When, how and why to make a therapeutic intervention?
5. Their view of how therapeutic intervention brings about change?

How do these two theories contrast with the short-term dynamic approach to the neuroses?
1. How does the clinical picture of the neurotic with oedipal conflict differ from the personality disorders with preoedipal arrest?

2. How do you make the differential diagnosis?
3. How do the therapeutic interventions differ?
4. How does the way the therapeutic interventions bring about change differ?

To anchor the discussion in clinical data rather than in abstract theoretical notions, we presented on the first day a discussion of three clinical case histories of psychotherapy of Personality Disorders, described by S. B. Nagel, Ph.D., R. Klein, M.D., and K. Clark, Ph.D., all of the Masterson Institute. In addition, P. Sifneos, M.D., gave a lecture on the short-term dynamic approach to the neuroses. On the second day, the Masters each had a three-hour workshop which allowed them to elaborate on their individual approaches. The conference concluded with a final hour and a half of panel discussion. The book follows the same format, thus allowing the reader to make his or her own clinical evaluation of the cases presented and then compare it with that of the experts.

The quality of the conference and of this book derives from the contribution made by the pioneering experts. Each had originated, developed, fought for, and expanded his or her own approach, which has stood the test of time and found a secure niche in the marketplace of ideas.

James F. Masterson, M.D., pioneered the developmental, object relations approach to the psychotherapy of the personality disorders through clinical research over the last 30 years. He is the founding father of the Society of Adolescent Psychiatry, Adjunct Clinical Professor of Psychiatry, Cornell University Medical College, and founder and director of the Masterson Institute, a nonprofit organization, and the Masterson Group. The body of Dr. Masterson's work is presented in the many books he has written, including the latest edited by him and Dr. Klein, *Psychotherapy of the Disorders of the Self: The Masterson Approach.*

Marian Tolpin, M.D., is a well-known writer and lecturer on self psychology who studied and collaborated with Heinz Kohut. Her original work on normal development poses major theoretical challenges to object relations approaches to clinical practice. Her current work on the unmirrored self includes fresh challenges to prevailing views on the psychology of women and men. Dr. Tolpin is a Training and Supervising Analyst at The Institute of Psychoanalysis, Chicago; an editor of *The Annual of Psychoanalysis* and of *Progress in Self Psychology*; and a founder and faculty member of The National Council for Psychoanalytic Self Psychology.

Peter E. Sifneos, M.D., is internationally known for his pioneering work on short-term dynamic psychotherapy. He is currently Professor of Psychiatry, Harvard Medical School, Associate Director in the Department of Psychiatry at Beth Israel Hospital in Boston, a practicing psychoanalyst, and Editor-in-Chief of *Psychotherapy and Psychosomatics*. He has done extensive research, writing, and teaching on the subject, as well as leading numerous workshops in Europe and North America. Dr. Sifneos is the author of *Short-Term Psychotherapy and Emotional Crisis* and *Short-Term Dynamic Psychotherapy: Evaluation and Technique.*

The book attests to the fact that the conference achieved its aim. The focus on detailed clinical material brought out clearly the differences in theory and technique. Often this type of conference produces bitter ad hominem attacks that clarify nothing. We were successful in avoiding this and in being able to disagree without being disagreeable. Hopefully, we have clarified the issues for the reader.

Following are the members of the Faculty of the Masterson Institute, who helped plan and present this conference:

James F. Masterson, M.D., *Director* Candace Orcutt, Ph.D., *Assoc.*
Ralph Klein, M.D., Cl. *Director* Karla Clark, Ph.D.
Richard E. Fischer, Ph.D., *Assoc.* Shelley B. Nagel, Ph.D.

PART I

Case Presentations and Discussions

1

Psychotherapy of a Lower-Level Borderline Personality Disorder

Shelley Barlas Nagel, Ph.D.

CASE PRESENTATION

Introduction

Kate was an articulate, intelligent, and charismatic 34-year-old single woman with a master's degree. I saw her in treatment for four and a half years. She was referred by her physician; the chief complaint was depression. During our work together, major treatment issues involved her self-destructive behavior, including a suicide attempt, volatile rage, and several serious addictions.

Presenting Information

At the time of her first appointment, Kate had been out of work for six months, supporting herself with money from a trust fund. A series of unsuccessful jobs finally ended when she was fired from her last position because she had come to work with her speech slurred from tranquilizers. She hated her work and wanted to change careers, but had no idea what she really wanted to do.

She felt depressed and lost, blaming her family, previous employers, and former lovers and therapists. Kate said sadly, "I'm tired of waking up depressed and scared. Outwardly, I'm pretty and charming. Inside, there's nothing. I hate myself."

Family History

Kate was the youngest and least favored of four children from a wealthy East Coast family. Her father, a graduate of an Ivy League school, was a prominent attorney. She described him as brilliant, but also remote, cold, and angry. He blamed Kate, not the other children, for his problems. She felt hated by him, even as she craved his attention.

Kate described her mother, a housewife and former model, as overpowering, critical, and controlling. "She demeaned me as a human being." Kate's mother had significant periods of depression and often used Kate as a scapegoat. Angrily, Kate said, "I hate my parents because now I have to rebuild my insides."

Past History

Kate's memory of her childhood was one of feeling sad, lost, and alienated. In first grade, despite her intelligence, she was held back because of poor concentration arising from anxiety and depression. She had few interests and no hobbies. Thirty pounds overweight in grammar school, Kate continued to fluctuate in weight most of her life.

In high school, however, she lost weight and became a gregarious school leader. She earned good grades with little effort, but underneath the facade she felt a gnawing sense of hopelessness, self-hate, and anger. To deaden these feelings, she smoked marijuana, drank alcohol, and experimented with drugs such as PCP, cocaine, and LSD. This drug use continued into her late twenties. She also took amphetamines to control her weight and to give her a high; she used Valium and Miltown to "take the edge off."

After failing the first semester at an out-of-state school, she returned home and attended a community college. Two years later, she moved away, finished her bachelor, and earned a masters degree. During this time, Kate had many brief and painful relationships with men. She was attracted to men who were emotionally unavailable, married, or abusive. Her longest relationship was with a heroin addict and drug dealer with whom she lived on and off for seven years. She went from job to job, being fired or quitting. Following graduate school, Kate had two abortions. She was raped a week after the second one.

She sought help with several therapists. The last, a psychiatrist, prescribed the antidepressant Norpramin, which Kate said never helped her. She told me that she had been drinking for many years and that her drinking and drug use had been ignored in all of her previous treatments whenever she had alluded to this behavior. Experiencing despair, rage, and self-hate, she had harbored recurrent thoughts of suicide most of her life. In fact, Kate had made five suicide attempts, the most serious occurring a year before she began treatment with me. After taking an overdose of Norpramin, she spent several days in an intensive care unit, barely managing to survive.

Treatment

Over the course of treatment, consisting of twice-a-week sessions, Kate discharged her feelings through behavior, not words. She defended against depression by using drugs and alcohol. She turned to men to take away her pain and to make her feel good. She went on massive eating binges and gained weight. She became bulimic, taking laxatives and diuretics while alternately bingeing and starving. She also acted out her rage by picking fights with coworkers and friends or by attacking me.

Kate needed to experience congruent, consistent treatment to help strengthen her reality perception, her ability to trust, and her sense of self. In the beginning of treatment, Kate tested me by missing appointments, arriving late, wanting me to see her on holidays, and asking me to prolong her sessions. Her payments were delayed and some of her checks bounced. She urged me to lower my fees and asked me to accept her as a non-paying patient when she lost a job. She tried to engage me in personal conversation, wanting our relationship to be personal rather that professional. When I did not comply with Kate's requests, but asked her instead to explore what prompted them, she attacked me for not caring.

Kate acted and reacted without thought of the consequences of her behavior. She wanted a quick fix—to numb and deaden her feelings. After an eating binge or a drinking episode, she felt remorseful and depressed, but continued her destructive cycle through further abuse of drugs and food. Each episode eroded her self-respect and self-image and reinforced her self-hate.

I can only speculate, based on my own work with patients with addiction problems, that Kate may have experienced physical and/or sexual abuse as a child. Childhood abuse appears to create a vulnerability to later problems with addiction. She had no clear memories of such abuse, but her intense acting out served to block many feelings and early memories.

From a neutral, yet empathic, stance, I brought to Kate's attention what she was not aware of: destructive behaviors harmful to her best interests. I made her present behaviors unacceptable to her by introducing conflict into her defensive system. At the basis of my confrontations was the conviction that Kate had the capacity to think, to stop herself from acting on impulse, to contain her feelings and talk about them in the sessions, and to act in a self-supportive manner.

By identifying her addictive and self-destructive behaviors, I followed the basic principle that priority be given to the process of stopping such actions—an issue that takes center stage in this type of treatment. Kate's patten of compulsion, loss of control, and continued abuse in spite of adverse consequences from drugs, alcohol, and food were addictions that could result only in a downward spiral. I confronted Kate's denial of her drug use. I asked, "Why are you hurting yourself with drugs and seeking an artificial high? I'd think you'd want to experience what you're feeling and be aware of your problems so that you could then solve them." Gradually, she internalized these questions and began asking them herself. She threw the amphetamines away. "I'm sick of the struggle," she said. But when she went through a period of withdrawal, she became depressed again and increased her drinking and use of tranquilizers.

Kate denied that alcohol was a problem, claiming, "I only take a few drinks. It makes me feel good. After all, I'm just a social drinker." I further confronted her denial by pointing out she had lost a number of jobs because of her drinking. Eventually, she showed signs of identifying with my perceptions and of integrating my confrontations by making efforts to cut back. Then, the arena of her conflicts shifted, and she engaged in a variety of defensive behaviors, including overeating, compulsive shopping, and verbal attacks on me.

Kate said to me, "I'm mad at you, I'm mad at this therapy. I feel like I'm under a microscope." Confronting the projection by putting it back in her head, I said "You have some choices: You can face your problems and feel some pain or you can deny your problems and dump your anger on me." She responded, "Looking at myself is hard. It's easier to focus on you, but I guess that doesn't help me much." "Right," I echoed.

I made it clear to Kate that using alcohol and drugs was at odds with coming to therapy. I said, "If you take alcohol for your pain, then you can't use treatment." I wondered if she had thought of going to Alcoholics Anonymous. She angrily responded, "That is the most obnoxious idea I've ever heard. Those people are disgusting creeps, and I'm mad you brought it up." I answered, "I don't know why you're getting so upset.

You've told me of your problems with drugs, your years of drinking, the loss of control, the blackouts and hangovers, the preoccupation and remorse. I'd think you'd want help." One of the main focuses throughout Kate's treatment was encouraging her participation in Alcoholics Anonymous—a necessary and important adjunct to her psychotherapy. Therapy alone would not be sufficient to manage her addictions. I did not see very much hope for her recovery without her involvement in AA.

Several weeks after she began treatment, Kate started attending AA meetings. At first, she had several bouts of drinking coupled with a few days of sobriety, followed by rationalizations, excuses, and attacks on AA. Then came efforts at self-control and limited drinking, but the limited drinking eventually gave way to heavy drinking. Kate ultimately realized that once she began drinking she could not stop. She hit bottom emotionally and she became hopeless and despairing. But, with her improved reality perception of these problems and their destructive consequences, she began to view her drinking and drug use as intolerable and unacceptable. She now turned to AA and to her therapy sessions to deal more honestly with her painful feelings about herself and her past.

At the same time, I was also confronting her lack of self-activation regarding her career. I said, "I'm wondering how it is you're not taking steps to look for work, so that you could have some structure to your days. I know it's a painful time, but you go to bed rather that push yourself to take some action that would make you feel better about yourself, instead of worse." I stressed her lack of functioning. Coping was crucial.

My confrontations and Kate's attempts at self-activation stirred up her depression and feelings of helplessness. Now she wanted me to take care of her and make things easy so that she would not have to take responsibility for herself. She said, "I can't do this, I don't know what to say next. Can't you help me and give me some direction?" I avoided resonating with her projection by not being drawn into the role of caretaker. With the underlying expectation that she could manage herself, I asked, "I'm wondering why you're feeling so helpless. How is it you feel you're not able to generate your own direction?" She said, "I can't do it. I feel so alone. The loneliness is unbearable." She started to cry, expressing despair.

After several months of sobriety, she talked about losing her sense of self when she was around her family. She said, "When I get around my family, I get so disoriented and doubtful about myself. I can't fight them." I asked her why she had such trouble supporting herself. She answered, "I need to figure out a way of being myself against them or how to process their input. I always got real depressed and would use drugs when my sisters and mother would say the family would really love me if I'd only open my heart. It was always as if I were the problem. Lately, I've had to shut down to come to grips with it." I pointed out that shutting down wasn't coming to grips with it. She responded, "I feel overwhelmed, and I start wondering if I'm crazy."

I suggested that, under her family's negative input, she conceded her judgment of reality to them, rather than sticking to her own. She replied, "My heart tells me if I don't protect myself against them, I'll end up dead. If I expose myself to them, I'll doubt myself. If they were in here, they'd swear they loved me." I answered, "You keep switching from your reality perception to their distortion as if it were reality." She answered, "It's hard to see the truth." She began crying and said, "I feel so uncomfortable talking to you about my family. I think you think I'm crazy or don't believe me." I answered, "You have been talking about giving up your own reality perception to your family's perception. Now you're doing the same thing. You think I'll see you the same way your family saw you. Do you notice you're doing this now with me?"

Kate began to see a relationship between her feelings and her behavior and to observe herself. Her self-image gradually improved, but, in reaction to her positive feelings, she criticized and attacked herself. She said, "I'm a jerk . . . spoiled . . .

nothing but a failure." I responded, "You were just acknowledging your pride in your efforts, and now you're attacking yourself. You call yourself names and beat up on yourself, rather than attempt to understand the way you feel." She started to acknowledge her positive efforts. But, her compassionate acknowledgment triggered feelings of anger and she then attacked me, accusing me of criticizing her. Reflecting her projection, I asked, "How is it you don't experience what I'm saying as being helpful? Instead, you think I'm attacking you. I'm pointing out how what you do in your life doesn't support you. How is that criticism?" She replied, "I guess what you say is helpful, but it's painful; being nice to myself is just not familiar." Again she wept and said, "The vicious attacks in my head are from my mother; that's how she talked to me." Kate expressed a sense of betrayal and sadness that her mother did not protect her from her father's abusive taunts, choosing instead to side with him against her.

After a year and a half of treatment, Kate's functioning had improved markedly. She no longer worked at minumum wage jobs beneath her ability. She relied more on herself, rather than on others. In her sessions, she was dealing with her feelings, not testing me as much or making me the target of her rage. She showed signs of treating me as an ally, rather than as an adversary, illustrating the strengthening of the therapeutic alliance.

But as she relied more on herself, she also felt depressed. She said, "I'm feeling worse than I've ever felt in my life." I replied, "Yes, I know you're feeling worse. It's because, as you're controlling your behavior, you're actually feeling more." I told her, "For you, feeling worse is good, not bad. Before, when you were using drugs and alcohol, turning to men, using sex to numb your feelings, and hating yourself, there wasn't any hope. You weren't going anywhere except down. You've been miserable most of your life. Now there's some purpose to your pain. Now it's possible to get to the bottom of it and to resolve your conflicts."

Kate mourned the wasted years of self-abuse and cried over the painful relationships with her parents and the love and support she had missed. She viewed her family with increasing clarity. She talked openly about her feelings of being left out as the unloved and least favored child. Kate saw her mother more realistically as a woman with emotional problems of her own and began to realize that she herself was not the cause of all her family's problems. She saw that her chaotic behavior and acting out were ways to hurt herself and were often compulsive, ritualistic repetitions of actual childhood scapegoating situations. However, after two or three sessions where she expressed sadness and rage about the past, she came to her sessions completely detached, with little memory of the previous sessions. I confronted the detachment by saying, "When you cut off feelings, you remove the possibility of being able to work them out." After tracking for several months this pattern of affect followed by detachment, I had to accept that Kate was not able to consistently experience feelings of rage, anxiety, and depression associated with self-activation and separation experiences without at times being overwhelmed. She intermittently lost the ability to think and to observe herself, and she detached affect. She returned to food binges and withdrew from her friends and AA.

In order to help Kate handle these feelings, I created a more supportive, focused therapy environment and turned from the goal of working through to the goal of ego repair during once-a-week sessions. Kate further developed the ability for self-observation and introspection. She realized that she was resisting the responsibility of growing up, a process that she associated with feelings of self-loathing, loneliness, and hopelessness. As time progressed, she identified with my perception of her as a competent, worthwhile person. However, the pattern of shifting behaviors continued, although to a much lesser degree. Kate initiated steps to activate herself positively, but then often retreated into despair; yet, she eventually came out of it. She learned to utilize concrete methods of coping with her depression. She listened to music and AA tapes, attended meetings, and maintained a long list of positive activities to do when she felt bad. And as time went on, the plunges into despair were shallower and lasted for shorter periods. She was better able to tolerate anxiety and to use anxiety as a signal to engage in self-supportive action rather than as a disorganizing, regressive pull toward addictive and self-destructive behavior.

Feeling more alive, Kate started to exercise and joined a running group. She felt closer to her friends and developed a caring circle of people around her. She pursued another graduate degree leading to a profession about which she had always secretly dreamed. Kate did not remain long in this positive space, however. Approaching her third year of sobriety in AA, she attended fewer meetings. Her on-and-off struggles with overeating took center stage in the treatment. She went on massive food binges. She gained weight and said that she hated herself. I confronted her impulsiveness and her pulling back from AA. I explored her feelings and tracked the sequence of events that led from her recent accomplishments and positive feelings to the destructive bingeing. Increasingly desperate, she started attending Overeaters Anonymous meetings.

Wanting neither to tolerate the bodily discomfort she experienced from overeating nor to face the consequences of her weight gain, she took laxatives and diuretics following the binges. Again, I confronted her destructive patterns, focusing on the compulsive overeating. In response, Kate said, "I don't want to give up this last problem; food and weight. Food protects me from feelings I don't want to face. I don't want to be totally healthy. What's more, I'm scared to death of a relationship with a man. Every time I get close to my goal weight, I get panicky because I feel terrific about myself—sexy and alive. Men look at me and want to be with me and I feel petrified. I want a relationship, but I keep sabotaging myself."

I explored her fears of closeness and of sexual intimacy and investigated her feelings of not wanting to be healthy. I pointed out the danger of taking laxatives and diuretics, but she denied their destructiveness. I insisted, "You are destroying yourself." She replied, "The destructive part of me doesn't want to give it up. It's familiar. It's part of me. I don't want to go through the pain. I can't stop." I said, "Saying 'I can't' is not accurate. You refuse." Kate answered, "Giving up crutches is frightening. Then, I'd have to turn to myself and I'm scared. I don't want to give it up. My mother doesn't deserve for me to get better. By my having problems and struggling, I'm hurting her. I have this personality that won't forgive." Noting the tenacity of her revenge fantasy, I asked, "Do you want to get back or do you want to get better? You can't do both." She answered, "I want to get better, but by staying the way I am, I want to get back. I know I have to get in touch with what's inside of me."

She tried to stop bingeing and to end her use of laxatives and diuretics. While Kate felt discouraged and struggled with the Overeaters Anonymous program, I gave her repeated encouragement. I reminded her that the "three steps forward and one step back" pattern was just part of the recovery process, as she well knew from her initial experience in recovery from alcohol and drugs. After some months, she stopped taking laxatives and diuretics and she followed a plan to eat three meals a day, with no eating in between. She also resolved not to take the first compulsive bite of foods she had repeatedly binged on.

Over the next several months, although Kate continued her cyclical pattern of success and despondency, the fluctuations were less intense and she followed through with her commitment to lose weight, no longer using food as a drug. But, even more important was her commitment to value herself by being in touch with her inner world. At this point in the treatment, Kate had come a long way from the time she began. She now had a stronger ego and a healthier self. She had an improved self-image and a better capacity for reality perception and self-expression. She was steadily employed at a job she found satisfying. She had made some gratifying friendships and she was involved in both the Alcoholics Anonymous and Overeaters

Anonymous fellowships. She had maintained sobriety and had abstained from drugs for three and a half years, and she no longer thought of suicide as an option when she experienced despair.

Now after losing 40 pounds, she was within three pounds of her goal weight and she looked terrific. As she came into my office wearing a new outfit she loved—the size she had always wanted to be—she said, "I'm so excited! It's not that I'm without problems, but I have hope. I know I have a depression, an abscess inside me. There are certain times, like when people leave me, or I speak up, or I push myself to do well, it's as though a sharp nail pokes it and pus seeps out all over inside of me. It's then that I feel so awful, but I have your voice in my head and the AA steps and I make healthy choices. As long as I don't do anything to hurt myself at that moment, the bad feelings pass. I can't believe it's me talking about feeling good about myself. If it wasn't for therapy and AA, I'd probably be dead."

So began a precipitous termination. She ended therapy soon afterwards. She did not want to face the anxiety and depression she felt as a result of her success, which involved good feelings about herself and about her relationship with me. I did not see her for six months. Then three weeks ago Kate called and came in for a session. Although she had lost her job, she was still in graduate school, and she had continued to maintain her sobriety and hope. I know that her path is not an easy one and that she continues to have problems. However, she now has a track record of resiliency and of overcoming obstacles. I have every hope that she will continue to grow, to make healthy, self-supportive choices, and to value herself more as a worthy human being.

2

Discussion of the Lower-Level Borderline Personality Disorder

Dr. Masterson: We conceive of the problem with a lower-level borderline, unlike the higher-level, as the patient's inability to work through the abandonment depression, inability to contain the affect. The objective of the treatment is ego repair.

What do I mean by that? This patient's primitive mechanisms of defense all operate at the cost of reality perception. You have to view the ego structure of the borderline as similar to a piece of Swiss cheese with all these holes in it in terms of reality perception. These defenses cannot operate without suspending reality perception.

What the therapist does by confrontation is lend the patient his/her reality-testing capacity. The patient identifies and internalizes this, improves his/her own reality perception, and is then able to better control and contain the abandonment depression, allowing the self to individuate and emerge further.

The differences between transference acting out, transference, and therapeutic alliance are crucial to this approach. The task of treatment, as we see it, is to convert transference acting out into therapeutic alliance and transference.

Therapeutic alliance is a real object relationship between therapist and patient in which they agree to work together to help the patient improve through insight and better control. It is based on the capacities of both therapist and patient to see each other as whole, good, and bad at the same time, in reality.

Transference is not a real object relationship, but is where the therapist serves as a target upon which are projected the patient's infantile fantasies and conflicts. At the same time, however, the patient must recognize the independent reality existence of the therapist. In other words, in order to have a transference as defined in this fashion, you have to have a therapeutic alliance because, if you do not have the reality screen or framework against which to contrast your projections, how can you understand that they are projections?

In transference acting out, however, the patient alternately projects and acts out on the therapist these alternating self and object representations, without any awareness at the time of the independent reality existence of the therapist as a therapist. Therefore, the way we then perform the task of therapy, helping the patient convert transference acting out into transference and therapeutic alliance, is through the therapeutic technique of confrontation.

What we mean by confrontation is not the eyeball-to-eyeball kind of thing we used to have with the Russians, which required a lot of aggression. As a matter of fact, if you're confronting from your own aggression, you won't be successful. Patients are very used to this and pick it up right away.

What we do mean by confrontation is the bringing to the center of the patient's attention the denied, maladaptive consequences of his or her defenses. In the case of

Kate, which we are discussing, these are the addictions to alcohol and drugs and the acting out with men.

In this form of treatment, it is not only what you do that is important, but also what you avoid. Since you are not going to work through the abandonment depression, you want to avoid those therapeutic activities that draw the patient deeper and deeper into the transference and deeper into the depression, for example, through fantasies, dreams, tranference, memories. Now I don't mean that you don't allow the patient to talk about these things. You do. But unlike what will happen in intensive analytic therapy where you take all these up for systematic investigation, you do not do so in shorter-term confrontive psychotherapy.

The patient has to find some more adaptive way to deal with episodes of abandonment depression that arise with separation stress. My patient would describe it this way: "It's like being in the ocean with your foot on the botton and you see a wave coming and you have to learn to tread water until the wave passes." Each patient has his or her own idiosyncratic individual style for finding a better way to manage these episodes while containing the abandonment depression. Somebody might change, as this patient did, from alcoholism and drug use to jogging, tennis, playing chess, although not everybody who does those things does them for the same reasons.

I think this is an extremely effective form of treatment with the borderline. The duration of treatment varies enormously, depending on the severity of the patient's illness. Kate happens, I think, to be a severely impaired lower-level borderline and I could see her being in confrontive therapy for a very long time, as long as the therapist wasn't colluding with regression.

Dr. Tolpin: I feel that I have a big job here. Let me make my overall point first. This therapist offers herself and herself-object functions without knowing them in her language, that is, in the theoretical framework that she has learned. And the patient makes use of these. I think the self psychological point of view that I'd like to try to get across delineates them more specifically and makes them the focus of the treatment for a very specific reason. The patient's disorder is essentially a disorder of not having within herself the wherewithal—the psychological capacities, as we call those structures—to be a self-propelling, self-initiating person with goals and ambitions, able to make good use of her talents and abilities.

The goal of the treatment from a self psychological point of view is very compatible with Dr. Masterson's outlook, but what differs is the outlook on how that goal is accomplished. The goal is accomplished through an explicit awareness that the therapist is offering these self-object functions for internalization. One can facilitate this process by making use of the transference, but not in the way it has been used classically. It is only in the transference development—understanding what disrupts the transference, which is a repetition of the early pathological experiences that are formative in the personality, and what repairs it—that the transmuting internalizations take over the needed self-object functions and repair occurs.

Let me address directly some of the things Dr. Masterson said so that I can get across some of the differences in point of view.

The patient's psychological task is to acquire the inner capacities to be self-activating. The rage, the depression, the helplessness, the substance abuse, the anxiety, the wanting the quick fix, the repeated relationships that are abusive, and so forth are all manifestations of structural deficit, that is, of her internal lack of the capacities that she needs.

Now, I think the reason Dr. Masterson's work, as I understand it, evolved in the way it did is that he recognized completely that the "Your pa was bad, your ma was bad" approach does not foster recovery. It fosters what he is afraid of, which is a kind of view that "You do it for me, since I've been so abused." This simply perpetuates pathology.

The reason Kohut's fundamental discoveries had such an enormous impact was that there was a way out of this dilemma that previous theories had not offered. What you are doing, essentially, when you ask the patient, "Why are you helpless? Why aren't you more sure of yourself? Why aren't you more self-directed?" is akin to telling a starving man, first, that he's not hungry and, second, that he ought to go out and provide his own source of food.

The goal is reasonable. Why doesn't the patient reject this approach? Some patients will reject any approach and some will accept any approach. Kate doesn't reject this approach because she experiences what she needs to experience, which is that this therapist recognize her inner lack, no matter how she conceptualizes it. The therapist says this is not a person who has the wherewithal to structure herself. Dr. Nagel tells us that she said right at the beginning, three weeks into the therapy, that Kate needed borrowed structure. That's what Alcoholics Anonymous is, borrowed structure with a kinship tie with other people. In self-psychological terms, that means alter egos, twinships where you have something in common, a bond which will get you into a more cohesive experience, with something to rely on, than you have within yourself plus what is offered in the treatment. This is an implicit way of recognizing structural deficit, even if it isn't an explicit way.

The patient, Kate, has a severe disorder of self-cohesion, with more emphasis on the behavior simply because it is more manifest. The primary pathology is that the center, or core, of the personality does not hold together adequately. Neither of the poles of the self-organization— ambitions or ideals—are adequately developed to a level where they lead or direct the personality. Therefore, the patient cannot direct herself, neither through ambitions nor ideals. Neither parent was available for the kind of protein, if you will, that a kid can take in and make into his or her own psychological structure.

Self-object functions are multiple; they belong in a whole group of categories. However, the category that is especially missing in this patient consists of all those things that make you feel you're together, that make you feel you're real, that give you some feeling of vitality. The disorder is a severe disorder of self-cohesion characterized by significant lacks in self-regulating capacities.

What do people do who have these self-regulating deficiencies? Exactly what this young woman does.

The high school, a gang, a group of peers, all are powerful self-object function providers. Kate's high school friends are like the group now in Alcoholic Anonymous and we have seen that they had a temporarily beneficial effect on her. What does she do? After she is out of a milieu that provides some structure, she turns to substances, sex, and protracted relationships, no matter what they are, because something is better than nothing.

The attempt to fill a void within oneself where capacities are lacking is so difficult that it leads to a kind of despairing depression, not the kind of depression that can be helped in some people by antidepressants. However, we should not eliminate a role for medication; we do anything we possibly can to try to fill that structural deficit.

Dr. Masterson views clinging, wanting a quick fix, helplessness, lack of direction and initiative, and self-destructive activity as defenses. From a self-psychological point of view, all of these are evidence of the structural deficit. What Dr. Nagel says—"This is is self-destructive, your behavior is hurting yourself, you need to try to control it as much as you can while we're working together"—

does temporarily provide structure and invite the patient into the relationship.

That's the fundamental difference. There is no point in looking at these as defenses where "the patient refuses to help herself." She doesn't have that capacity now, but what she does have is the capacity to enter into a relationship which is not short-term. Dr. Masterson says you don't use the transference or what you can understand about the transference in short-term supportive therapy. This means four and a half years of therapy.

Understanding more about yourself and the patient in the room would lessen the exhortative, educational aspect and foster, I think, more possibility for internal reorganization, although some of that is certainly taking place here.

Dr. Sifneos: I have learned a great deal from the experts who use long-term therapy because I'm spoiled. The patients whom we treat are really healthy people with very circumscribed types of difficulties.

I would like to view this from a variety of points of view and raise questions as to whether, indeed, there is this great difference that Dr. Tolpin has just discussed between defensive and structural deficits.

First of all, I view this patient, Kate, as having a total anhedonia and alienation from the world. In terms of DSM III-R, she could be diagnosed as having a depression; there is a family history of depression. She could be diagnosed as being an addict; certainly, she has drug addiction and alcohol addiction. She can be diagnosed as suffering from bulimia nervosa or anorexia. All these tags add up to a diagnosis of severe borderline personality.

However, the anhedonia and the alienation are crucial. I am also impressed by Dr. Nagel's speculation as to whether there is a childhood trauma, possibly on a preverbal level, that this young lady was unable to express.

Therefore, she had to rely on support from the outside to fill in the basic gap.

Is this point of view different from Dr. Tolpin's? There is a structural deficit, a basic alienation, which has to be filled in by something. Therefore, Kate relies on a variety of ways that make her feel better temporarily: alcohol, sex, drugs, and food.

These are all self-destructive as far as we are concerned, thus creating the dilemma facing the therapist. They are self-destructive but they are the only things that keep Kate going. Otherwise, life would not be worthwhile.

So the therapist here is presented with a very difficult situation: the need to attack these things, to criticize them, to try to have the patient be different even while that patient rejects this approach because these ways of acting are all that she has known.

This is why I think she refuses AA at first with some very derogatory terms. But eventually, once she gets going with it and finds out there are other people in the same category as she is, anhedonic, alienated, then she begins to move in a positive way.

I'm intrigued here by one aspect which has something to do with what we do in shorter-term psychotherapy—namely, the focusing that Dr. Nagel has pointed out. She emphasized some of the positive activities that the patient was achieving. The patient denied it at first, but nevertheless continued having these positive activities. This means that slowly the therapeutic alliance was being established and she was willing to exchange some of the destructive things that she had been doing for a therapist who was the recipient of all these aspects.

Dr. Nagel, please don't get me wrong, but you were the drug, you were the LSD, you were the food, you were everything. Slowly, however, you started replacing these very malignant ways of being over a long period of time with yourself. And there we have in a sense the transference, the acting out transference that Dr. Masterson was talking about, becoming progressively an ego supportive, therapeutic alliance.

Once again I raise this question: Is there that much difference between these points of view? The behavior is defensive in the sense that Kate doesn't have the equipment for a while and, therefore, has to fill it in with something. In that sense, in my opinion, it is defensive.

Dr. Masterson: Let me first put together Dr. Tolpin's questions with Dr. Sifneos' comments. Dr. Tolpin's perspective is that the basic psychopathology is an injured self-cohesion. My perspective basically agrees that the patient has deficient capacities of the self.

The way I differ is that I see this injured self-cohesion as a product of a developmental arrest which springs from the need to defend against abandonment depression. In clinical terms, while Dr. Tolpin focuses on self-cohesion, I focus on that by implication as a consequence of the developmental arrest because of the abandonment depression.

Dr. Tolpin argues that the defenses are efforts at self-structure. I do not disagree with that because I see them as ways in which the patient keeps herself from feeling bad in the light of the fact that she doesn't have mature capacities of the self and she does have the abandonment depression to deal with.

I never say to a patient, as Dr. Tolpin stated, "Why are you helpless?" I say, "I wonder why you feel helpless." Huge difference. Dr. Tolpin's idea was that there is no point in saying to a person who is hungry and doesn't have food, "Why are you hungry and why don't you get food?" They can't do it. As if that's what we're doing when we say, "I wonder why you feel helpless?" This leads to a crucial distinction between the two points of view.

How do we expect this patient with the depression, the

defenses, and the lack of capacities of the self to benefit
from what we're doing? I think Dr. Sifneos has put his
finger on it. The therapist works from an implicit assumption that the patient does have that capacity—which can
be mobilized by appropriate intervention. The therapist
then identifies the defenses and points them out to the
patient, thus creating conflict over behavior which the patient considered ego syntonic. In other words he helps the
patient to change her perspective or her behavior from
ego syntonic to ego alien. And how does this happen? I
know that in self psychology it is called transmuting internalization. I would call it identification and internalization of the therapist functions with the patient through
the therapeutic alliance.

The confrontations deal not only with the defensive
behavior; they also deal with the projections on the therapist and help the patient to see the therapist as he is, to
take in the therapist perspective. This is what provides the
structure, fills those holes in ego function, and enables the
patient to begin to activate herself. The therapeutic alliance
and the internalizations that spring from it are a very powerful and crucial factor.

Finally, Dr. Tolpin mentioned that I don't use the transference. This is not what I said. I said we don't "work
through" the transference as we would in intensive analytic
therapy whose specific purpose is to work through the
transference. It becomes the center stage of treatment.

Dr. Tolpin: One of the significant changes for the treatment of
a broad spectrum of patients is the concept that understanding the transference is crucial, but in a different way
than previously. This is a transference where the patient
feels backed, supported, encouraged. The therapist is
hopeful for her, sees something in her, recognizes something, validates that something, has a sustaining, very

gentle, on her side quality. Those are self-object functions. That is a self-object transference.

There is no reason in the world why that kind of transference shouldn't be placed in the center and understood in terms of its disruptions. I would hazard the guess that some of the depressions and some of the behavior, if understood in terms of what disruption occurred and how that is repaired, might have been set to rights somewhat without so much falling apart and return to the methods of self-preservation.

This point of view about the transference and what its role is makes an enormous difference. Its role is essentially the role of people in normal development. Thus, if somebody is falling apart, you don't say, "Pull yourself together." Rather, you offer the helping hand, as it were. And that's essentially what this transference does. So the recommendation is to follow it, to talk about it out loud, to understand it with the patient, to explain it to the patient, and to look for what is disrupting it when the patient begins to fall apart or to become devitalized again. While one may think about the detachment as a defense, which often it is, it's also a sign of the devitalization of the personality.

The thing you don't hear very much in these presentations is the shame that is one of the bases for this patient's self-hatred. Kate doesn't have to be helped to make her behavior ego dystonic. She has to be helped to have the wherewithal so she doesn't have to resort to it. She is massively ashamed of herself.

Dr. Sifneos: Of course she is, but the question is why she is the way she is. We have to raise certain speculations about the causation of this particular problem. In my opinion, it is because, whatever the reasons, she had this inability in very early childhood and, therefore, feels different. I think you're right, Dr. Tolpin, when you say she might feel the shame. I, also, would feel ashamed if I descended from the moon and all of you were speaking in a different language. I would feel completely alienated. Therefore, I have to look for something that is going to make me feel better. And for a while I find some very easy, quick fixes: drugs, LSD, alcohol, and food.

What Dr. Nagel has done over a long period of time is to slowly and steadily make me feel a part of the planet earth. That's a tremendous achievement.

Dr. Masterson: I think Dr. Tolpin has put her finger on the crucial difference. As I understand what she is saying, the curative feature has to do with the management of the so-called self-object transference. My point is very different from that. I think that with borderline patients, Dr. Tolpin's approach runs into serious risks because it drastically diminishes the patient's reality perception and draws her into this world of fantasy and emotion.

I see the crucial therapeutic agent quite differently. All those positive supports for the self that you see coming from self-object transference cannot come from transference because transference exists not in reality but in fantasy, and the internalization of a fantasy doesn't lead to better reality adaptation. I try to help the patient see the distinction between transference and therapeutic alliance. In my view all of those positive supports for self-activation come from the therapeutic alliance and the therapist's support of self-activation at the same time that the therapist's confrontations are internalized.

Dr. Tolpin: Self-object transferences are real. Everybody learned in psychoanalytic training or from the derivatives of psychoanalytic training that transference is a distortion.

The healthy part of development that is remobilized in self-object tranferences contains valid developmental needs. I think Dr. Klein's case will bring out the difference between pathological aspects of the personality that are immoblized and valid developmental needs that are immobilized. Of course, the therapist has to understand the difference between what is pathological and what belongs to normal development.

I think the reason that following a transference was either futile or destructive for many patients and therapists was that the transference was understood in terms of mobilizing pathological structures that would be then endlessly repeated, both with the therapist and outside. The healthy part of the personality that needs backing and needs borrowed structure was not recognized as the center of the transference. That's what the transference is in Dr. Nagel's case. You would not say that Kate has a distortion when she experiences, and that's what keeps her going and that's what keeps her coming back and that's what enabled her to overcome the shame and go to AA and so forth. She experienced Dr. Nagel as a backer who is enthusiastic about her—one of the vital functions that she was missing in a childhood of abuse.

Dr. Masterson: But is that transference or is that real?

Dr. Tolpin: That's self-object transference and it's real.

Dr. Masterson: This is a new definition of transference. Usually it's thought of as a fantasy from the past projected into the present. What I call therapeutic alliance you call self-object transference.

Question: Dr. Nagel gave some very nice examples of interventions from the Masterson perspective and I'd be very interested in hearing from a self-psychology perspective how you would intervene differently with a clinging or helpless kind of response from the patient. Specifically, what would you say?

Dr. Tolpin: You've got to understand the differences in point of view before you start talking about this or that intervention. It's like starting to play a board game and not knowing any of the rules. The opening moves, as it were, belong to the basic orientation of the therapist, which is, in your terms, borderline, and in my terms, a very severe disorder of self-cohesion.

Of course, you don't ask the patient to lie on the couch and tell you about her childhood, right? And there's a very commonsensical element in Masterson that is enormously important. But that element itself is a therapeutic attitude that is loaded with the recognition of what this patient needs. So, one of the opening moves is that you tell her about that. Essentially, Dr. Nagel did that. You tell her that she needs more structure in her life, she needs more organization, she needs backing and support, and so forth, all of which she lacks. You also tell her, so as not to be overwhelming but at an appropriate time, that clearly she has abilities and you would think she could make more use of them.

Many of the things that Dr. Nagel has done would be appropriate to do from the idea of a self-object transference. How you look at this evolving situation is really crucial to what you're going to do about it. That is why there is some point to learning about clinical theory. What you think about it tells you what to do about it.

Question: Dr. Masterson, I was wondering if you could help me understand theoretically why a lower-level borderline can never learn to swim, why he always has to tread water when the waves wash over him.

Dr. Masterson: That's a difficult question to answer and will vary from case to case, but our working hypothesis is that the patient's capacities for the self and self-activation have been too damaged in early life to be fully repaired. There are other ways of saying it. They have been exposed to entirely too much abandonment depression and they do not have enough ego strength to work it through. I think, for example, Dr. Nagel chose the course of requiring that the patient demonstrate to her that she was unable to do it, which I think is the proper course to take.

Once you've made the decision that the patient cannot do it, then your therapeutic prospects are limited, as is your therapeutic approach, and so you put a ceiling on the patient's prospects until you've tested it out in the clinical arena to get the evidence to make your decision. You want to give the patient the benefit of the doubt in the beginning of treatment.

I think this is one of the advantages of our various theoretical approaches. The self psychologist would speak of the patient's self being too damaged to be able to be restored.

Dr. Tolpin: Yes and no. You know abandonment depression, incidentally, is Masterson's conceptualization of structural deficit. . . .

Dr. Masterson: And structural deficit is the self psychology conceptualization of an abandonment depression.

Dr. Tolpin: Right. It depends on which direction you're coming from. Every school of psychoanalytic thought has struggled with this, so it's a very valid point that we've all tried to describe.

Yes, there are different views about a self and its original outlines, what injuries were sustained, and what can be done. But they are different in this sense. First of all, the idea that the pathology necessarily has to be so early is not part of my version of self psychology, even though it's always understood that way. Second, there is no way of knowing until you have the trial of treatment.

That is why it is important to take your diagnosis with a grain of salt, not to add up the symptoms and say this means this and this means that. Otherwise, you can't be open to the enormous potential that exists when there is backing of a personality that has been so chronically unbacked and unsupported.

Dr. Nagel has encouraged the patient to take initiative and that's fine. The encouragement is important as long as it's understood that in some people's hands this could be called nagging. I could tell from Dr. Nagel's account that it is not. But it would be nagging or exhortation on the part of some therapists. It would be a pull yourself together kind of thing.

When the patient says, "I can't do it, I don't know what to say next, can't you help me and give me direction," Dr. Nagel's conception is that she has to avoid resonating with her patient's projection that she's so helpless.

Dr. Masterson: We call that the rewarding unit projection.

Dr. Tolpin: Okay. This is a defensive pattern that has to be interrupted. Because of Kate's helplessness and the secondary gain and so forth, Dr. Nagel doesn't want to be drawn into the role of the caretaker. She holds an underlying expectation that the patient could manage herself. Dr. Nagel says "I'm wondering why you're feeling so helpless. How is it you feel you're not able to generate your own direction?" Kate said, "I can't do it. I feel so alone. The loneliness is unbearable." She started to cry, expressing despair.

And then, because this is a process, after several months of sobriety she talks about losing her sense of self when she is around her family. She gets so disoriented and doubtful about herself. Okay, when the patient says, "Can't you help me and give me some direction?" I might say, "Yes, you feel helpless and unable to do it when you temporarily lose the feeling of the backing that you need. And so you turn to me, looking for support and encouragement and backing."

You might carefully ask some patients, "What happened that you feel less supported? Has something happened that you feel less supported?" You don't say, "I haven't supported you." This is not intended as blame for the therapist. Rather, the idea is that you have brought forward the possibility of backing. This patient has healthy needs for backing. If they are not adequately responded to, you may see a temporary setback, a further disruption, or a disorganization, the one step back after the three steps forward. And so you look at it with her.

Incidentally, the way alliance develops is through your understanding and explaining the transference. That is because much of what has been called therapeutic alliance is, in fact, real and it's a self-object transference. The patient finally feels she has an ally that she can work with, somebody who is attempting essentially to understand her and to explain it to her.

You see, my "Yes" doesn't say, "Yes, I'll give you a sense of direction." It doesn't say, "Yes, pull yourself together." It just says, "Yes." And then you explain exactly what it is that you understand about this temporary return to the experience of collapse, helplessness, and despair.

Dr. Masterson: When the patient asks, "Can't you help me," we view this as an expression of the helplessness about the self and a projection of the omnipotent object on the therapist to take over in a regressive fashion. And so we turn to the patient and say, "I wonder why it is that when you're feeling this way you turn to me. What makes you feel this way?" Then, the moment the patient starts to say, "I feel so alone," in my view this patient is at this point beginning the repair of the deficit in self-activation by being willing to focus work on the affect that prevents her from activating herself.

My concern about your view that you would say, "Yes," when the patient is projecting, not transference, but transference acting out, is as follows: When they do that, they don't see you as you are, but rather as a literal repetition of this infantile figure from the past. When you respond with, "Yes, I will do what you ask," that reinforces the rewarding projection and regresses the patient. This is reinforcing the past rather than helping the patient to deal with it.

In our experience with borderline disorders, this response is like pouring fuel on a fire. You just increase the need for support enormously. Then, what are you going to do the 16th time the patient says, "Can't you help me?"

You started off saying, "Yes," which I don't really agree with, but then you went on to say you felt bad, which is not terribly different from what we would say. But I think this points out this crucial difference between us: You say that transference cures, but in my terms you're talking about the therapeutic alliance and I maintain that it is the contrast between transference acting out and therapeutic alliance which cures.

Dr. Tolpin: We're not going to get a divorce because we've never been married, but we're going to go on struggling to communicate. There are people who think it's hopeless to try to translate from one theoretical framework into another. I am not one of them, but this is one of those times where it is difficult.

Dr. Masterson: This is what we call a self-object transference disruption.

Dr. Tolpin: The difficulty we're having arises from the fact that the assumptions underlying Dr. Masterson's point of view and my point of view are really incompatible. These assumptions have then determined everything else. When I say, "Yes," that's just an example of responding to the patient when she says, "Can't you help me?" If I say, "Yes," I wouldn't fault it because my "Yes" isn't, "Yes, I'm going to take care of you. Yes, I'm going to foster your being helpless." My "Yes" is responding temporarily to those needs that were immobilized and that help activate you when they're responded to. It's an exploratory intervention. It's an interpretive intervention. It is not your idea of a caretaking intervention, the "Honey, it's too bad," or, "Yes, I'll direct you." It isn't that kind of a "Yes."

Dr. Nagel's work shows you a coaching no. She says, "No, don't do that," "No, that isn't good for you," "No, I think you should do it this way." It isn't a malignant or undermining no. One might make a distinction between a malignant yes and a coaching yes. A malignant, undermining yes in your view and my view would be to foster some kind of helplessness that clearly isn't there in the personality.

Dr. Masterson: I think our disagreement here goes beyond therapeutic approach. It goes to diagnosis because, as I understand it, self psychology does not recognize the Borderline Personality Disorder as being different from the Narcissistic Disorder. Rather, self psychology sees this as just another variation of injured self-cohesion. Is that correct?

Dr. Tolpin: No, no.

Dr. Masterson: I know that self psychology uses the concept of "borderline," but what you seem to mean is "borderline psychotic." I'm not talking about that. I'm talking about a stable borderline personality structure. Does self psychology view it as Kohut originally described it—borderline psychotic who cannot be analyzed?

Dr. Tolpin: I'm happy to say there is no monolithic self psychology. The great thing about the Kohut contribution is that a number of people have been attracted to it and a great deal of work is going on in different directions with differences in views amongst them. That is the healthiest development that has taken place in psychoanalysis for many years, in my view.

My view is that borderline is a pejorative diagnosis. It is soaked in theories that I do not think adequately explain disorders of the self. Dr. Klein will give us an example, I think, of the harmful use of diagnosis in a hospital instance where there was some diagnostic rationalization, I'm certain, for what was being planned.

My view is that it would be much better to think of these disorders that have been called borderline as various kinds of severe disorders of self-cohesion, which you describe later in more detail with the test of treatment. There is no diagnosis in dynamic psychoanalytically oriented psychotherapy that can be made from a cluster of symptoms that does not do you and the patient an injustice. You do it as you go along and you have to think about it. You do not start out with a set diagnosis.

3

Psychotherapy of a Narcissistic Personality Disorder
(The First Two Years)

Ralph Klein, M.D.

CASE PRESENTATION

I saw John Rosen, 44, in a hospital consultation requested by the ward staff to evaluate the possible use of ECT. He had been hospitalized for the third time in the past year for depression and suicide gestures.

Upon questioning the staff, I found that the patient had no vegetative or melancholic symptoms to warrant such an action. In fact, though the patient stated that he was profoundly "depressed," there were almost no observations by the ward staff to support such a diagnosis. The patient interacted so well with the other patients that he had been elected patient representative at a recent community meeting. Why the consideration for electroconvulsive therapy?

Essentially, the staff was furious at this patient for frustrating all their efforts to help him. He seemed to "wallow in his misery" (as one staff member put it). He would start to feel better and become optimistic and excited with his progress, only to rapidly relapse and express profound sadness with himself and disappointment with the staff who were failing despite their best efforts—as he would remind them.

The entire milieu staff, from therapy aide to treating psychiatrist, felt alternately hopeful and good—and then increasingly frustrated, disappointed, disillusioned, and, finally, angry. The anger had been especially exacerbated by the results of a blood-level study for an antidepressant which the patient was taking. The test was done to evaluate whether the blood level of the drug was within a therapeutic range. The patient had not been told the purpose of this particular test. The test was done twice. The results had been the same both times. The blood level was zero. Review of procedures had uncovered only one possible explanation for the result—the patient was not taking the medication. Rather than raise this matter with the patient, the staff decided to pursue the possibility of ECT.

The initial meeting took place at a ward clinical case conference. The patient was informed that I was an expert consultant who would decide what further treatment course should be followed. While the patient, who was quite verbal and articulate, provided much interesting information during the conference, the most striking impression I had then—and which I have only very infrequently experienced since—was the patient's sense of excitement, of eager expectation that talking with me would provide him the "magical answers" to his problems. He recounted his hopes with all the intensity and characteristics of a prayer and he concluded his comments in the evaluation with the statement that he was hopeful that either I, or God, would hear his plea and help him. At the time, I recall feeling that he was making no distinction between the two and that I was uncomfortable with the intensity of his idealization and his need for "perfect understanding" or "mirroring."

The patient's past history was further revealing. He described a basically unhappy childhood, yet with feelings of being special at the same time. He attributed this largely to his being the youngest of three children (the closest sibling was nine years older). He remembered his mother as a particularly self-centered and dependent woman. The father was recalled as spending little time with the children, but as someone whom he admired and with whom he loved spending time. He later recalled that the time with the father established a pattern repeated thoughout his life—of eager expectation which was rarely realized and was therefore, followed by profound and angry disappointment. One particular memory of childhood seemed to exemplify this. He would love to visit his father's factory with him on weekends and was thrilled at what seemed to be the vastness of the building and his father's importance. However, one weekend, upon leaving through a rear doorway, the patient recalled seeing several "bums" living in the alley behind the factory. He recalled being quite frightened, aware that his father could not protect him if the men tried to harm him, and he never subsequently wanted to (nor did he) return to the factory.

His father died when the patient was 10. He recalled that at the time his primary feeling was not of sadness, but of emptiness. He thought he remembered this clearly as, "How could he do this to me?" Later in treatment, Mr. Rosen was to recall that his mother's reaction was essentially the same and that she was unavailable to him because of her own self-involved preoccupations. The sense the patient conveyed was of a childhood in which there was no reliable figure to serve as a consistent source of soothing, calming, values, or ideals, and, hence, of a stable, cohesive sense of self—especially a sense of self-worth, self-esteem and well-being.

Mr. Rosen characterized his adolescence as dominated by two themes: First was the feeling that he could get whatever he wanted and achieve the success he desired by doing only a minimum of work, only what was required of him, no more, no less. Although he did not express it as such at the time, this theme seemed to reflect his feeling that the way to receive narcissistic supplies was to mirror precisely the expectations of others—no more, no less. The second theme was his obsessive concern with the size of his penis, which he felt was inordinately small and a constant source of shame and of potential humiliation by friends and girls. His penis was, among other things, a metaphor for his underlying fragmented, empty, vulnerable self.

The patient had attended college, where he got a degree in engineering. He married his first wife on the day he graduated because, "I wanted to have someone who could take care of my needs." He began to be moderately successful in his career and had two children within the first few years of marriage "to prove that I could, that I was a man." However, he felt constant discontent. He was constantly living beyond his means and always felt that he had to have a better car, a better and bigger house, and, finally, a better and more satisfying wife and life. He stated he became quite depressed at this point, made a suicide gesture, and proceeded to enter psychotherapy. Treatment consisted of eight sessions with a therapist who "convinced me that the solution to my depression lay in divorce." The patient left his family (after 15 years of marriage) and took up a bachelor's life. His depression lifted almost immediately.

At first, he was happy with his "new life" and continued to do well professionally while dating frequently and having "good sex" for the first time. He got involved in a social network, supported by a church, for single and divorced adults and became president of the organization. It was here that he met his future second wife. Approximately 18 months prior to my consultation, the patient had experienced a series of misfortunes. First, he was asked to leave the group that he was president of when it was discovered that he was "borrowing" money from the organization's treasury. This involved several thousand dollars, but no charges were pressed and the patient justified the behavior as appropriate reward for the work he put in. Mr. Rosen immediately married the woman he had been involved with. However, the relationship rapidly deteriorated as he experienced sexual difficulties (episodic impotence and premature ejaculation) and intense "competitive feelings" toward his new wife's two children. Lastly, his immediate boss at work, a man whom he admired and who admired him, had retired and a new boss had taken over. He had been hospitalized three times, all briefly, for suicidal ideation and, most recently, for a suicide gesture in which he stabbed himself in the chest superficially with a letter opener.

Course of Treatment: The Initial Phase

Following my initial evaluation of the patient, I recommended that no ECT be given and that the patient be discharged to outpatient therapy with a recommendation for intensive psychotherapy. The staff took my suggestion and discharged the patient, who called me for treatment. I saw him twice weekly for the first year and then three times per week.

Initially, the patient presented with a continuation of the theme of depression and hopelessness. There seemed to be a multitude of suicidal ideas and vague threats: sleeping with scissors under his pillow in case he got the desire or courage to stab himself; trying on several occasions to put a plastic bag over his head to see what it would feel like to suffocate; fantasizing about throwing himself on the subway tracks while waiting for a train. However, there was never a sense of real depression on his part or real concern on my part. Rather, this theme seemed clearly to serve as a distraction to keep him from focusing on real concerns and conflicts. It was also an effort to shift the focus of the sessions to what I would do to "rescue" him. I would repeatedly interpret to him that it was so painful for him to expose himself and his real concerns in treatment that he felt the need to protect himself by his obsessive preoccupation with self-harm.

Such interpretations would usually result in brief insights and interruptions in his defense.

For example, Mr. Rosen would reflect and then respond that maybe he *was* using these ideas as an escape. Maybe, he would add, it was a way of latching on to an identity when he didn't like the identity that he saw when he really looked at himself. He would then typically pause and reflect that he didn't like the feelings this brought up—that he began to feel excited that I understood him and could help him, but he knew that it was only a matter of time until he became disillusioned in me, too. I would then reflect that it was so painful for him to focus on himself that in order to protect himself he would feel the need to turn to me for answers. Then he was disappointed when I didn't respond as he felt or wished I would.

Again, defense would briefly give way to reflection: "At times it feels like I just move from one fantasy to another. It's discouraging. I know that the feeling is that I want more from you. It feels like I need protection from these thoughts and that you will promise to help and then just disappoint me." I would reflect, typically, that it is so difficult to look at what you want or can do with yourself that you protect yourself by focusing on the things you hope to get from me.

He would again think and respond: "It *is* difficult to look at myself. Sometimes when I meet people, I don't know what to call myself. I feel so insecure, embarrassed. As if I can't grasp myself. It feels like all my thoughts and feelings are illegitimate. I *guess* I don't feel good about me. There is not much self-respect. I *guess* there is not much to respect and admire."

As Mr. Rosen spoke of these feelings early in the treatment, I noted that his feelings of illegitimacy were conveyed without much emotional tone or turmoil, while his pronouncements of diminished self-respect and self-worth were tentative: he "guessed" and "supposed" this was how he felt. I felt that he was trying to be a good patient and say what he thought I wanted to hear. In short, I felt he was trying to mirror my expectations and needs so that I would provide narcissistic supplies in return.

As I continued to interpret his difficulties in focusing and concentrating upon himself, a new theme began to emerge around the third month of treatment. As his obsessive ruminations diminished and he became more convinced of my willingness and ability to listen to him noncritically, he began to reveal the underlying fantasies beneath the manifest level of self-attack. In fact, rather that his self-attacks (verbally and physically) reflecting self-loathing, they reflected quite the opposite. He revealed more and more that his suffering was ennobling and reflected his belief that he was actually first among God's chosen—a Job-like figure whose capacity to endure would actually be a source of enormous envy to those who recongnized it. In fact, his favorite self-representation was that of Saint Sebastian and he kept several pictures of St. Sebastian in his home—pictures that portrayed Sebastian tied to a stake with a multitude of arrows piercing him. Along with the emergence of this theme came the further understanding of his feelings of never having to do more than the minimum in order to get narcissistic supplies. Essentially, he felt that his suffering more than sufficed to entitle him to have all he wished.

Self-aggrandizement, therefore, was the second level of defense beneath the level of self-attack and rumination. This manifestation of his grandiose self was far more pervasive and central to his conscious self-identity and far more central as a basic protective armor keeping his real, vulnerable, fragmented, and empty self out of awareness.

Mr. Rosen's self image as the Perfect Martyr now moved to center stage in the psychotherapy and became the focus of the interpretations about, and the exploration of, his narcissistic vulnerability. I would repeatedly interpret that it was so painful for him to focus on the bad feelings about himself that in order to restore his sense of self he turned to invest emotions in others and to try to be the Perfect Martyr in their eyes. Slowly, he would begin to acknowledge this and to eleaborate on his extreme sensitivity to others and the need to be the Perfect Martyr in their eyes. This unleashed anger and depression which he defended against by acting out primarily through helplessness. The patient's chronic difficulties in functioning, which had typically been attributed to "depression," increasingly gave way to a more complicated, narcissist explanation. It took on

the characteristics of a "sit down strike" in which the patient
would wait for someone or something to come along and "rescue" him from his loneliness, stagnation, and emptiness.

Interpretations of these defenses against narcissistic vulnerability led to further exploration: "People will laugh at me if I
am not the Perfect Martyr." Also, "I feel depressed and confused. I feel lost. How do I handle myself without being the
Perfect Martyr? Whenever I felt that it wasn't working, I would
get depressed and that is when I would want to kill myself or
just run away, like I guess I have been doing most of my adult
life." This exploration led to more defense: "What else is there?
Right now I feel angry at myself. I have those old feelings again
of wanting to hurt myself." I interpreted that he invested so
much emotion in the image of the Perfect Martyr and in pro-
tecting the good image of others (especially his parents, as I
understood it) that his anger had no place to go and so was
reflected back on himself.

These interpretations slowly took hold and he returned to
the memory of the loss of his father at age 10 and then to other
memories that went back even further to his feelings of profound humiliation, fear, and loss starting when he was very
young. These were associated with his mother's lack of acknowledgment (due to her own self-preoccupation) and his
father's lack of availability—feelings which were expressed in
the prototypic experience in his father's factory at the age of
seven which emotionally was felt as desertion by both mother
and father.

However, this led to further resistance as he needed to deny
the longing left unfulfilled by the feelings of desertion. At these
times, he would reassert his intense envy of anyone who was
successful and his absolute insistence would emerge that he
was entitled to like success, without hard work. For example,
in his relationships his fantasy was that "a beautiful woman
would see me on the street, realize that I was what she had
always been looking for all her life, and she would approach
me, want me, appreciate me, and take care of me."

I dealt with these resistances by clarification of his struggle between the grandiose self and his emerging real self. I interpreted his fantasies of entitlement as related to his anxiety about growing up, focusing on his real feelings and on his giving up the Perfect Martyrdom while supporting himself.

At this point, some two years into treatment, Mr. Rosen began to tentatively explore the rage and depression of his fragmented self. The fragmented self had several levels that were associated with and represented by his feelings of desertion, his feelings of sexual inadequacy (i.e. his small penis), and his underlying self-image as a "derelict" and a "bum." All had to be worked through in the treatment, both in relationship to the past and in the mirroring transference acting-out in the sessions. I would interpret his mirroring defense in the treatment as I had his Perfect Martyrdom defense as a way to manage and soothe the painful feelings of rejection, inadequacy, and emptiness experienced about himself which were impelled by my therapeutic neutrality. This issue required much work in the course of the treatment.

The treatment of this patient was long and arduous. There were a multitude of secondary themes, conflicts, distortions, and defenses which had to be dealt with. Throughout the treatment, however, the main emphasis was on narcissistic vulnerability—i.e., how painful it was to focus on the self and the patient's need for idealizing and mirroring defenses against this vulnerability as manifested in his grandiose self and his Perfect Martyrdom, along with the secondary features of entitlement, envy, sexual inadequacy, and the sit-down strike, among others. The focus on narcissistic vulnerability in and out of the transference acting-out led to working through of depression and anger and the emergence of his real self from behind the shadow of St. Sebastian and Job. His life became more adaptive, as manifested by realistic striving and genuineness in his relationships such that people became real, independent centers of initiative rather that mere shadows or mirrors.

4

---

*Discussion of Psychotherapy
of the Narcissistic
Personality Disorder*

Dr. Tolpin: I can see from this case history why there's a flirtation. We seem to be talking the same language and then suddenly we're not. The way that Dr. Klein describes many of the characteristics of displaced development, the way he sees the unavailability of solid consistency of either a mother and father, his description of the vulnerable, empty feeling, fragmented self—we're both using the same language. And then the flirtation ends in trouble because we're going down different theoretical outlooks that have enormously affected what is considered defense, what is considered the primary pathology, and how you intervene with it.

Let me stay with the more diagnostic considerations. This is a moderately severe disorder of the self, characterized by overt pathological grandiosity and hidden pathology of ideals. The overt pathological grandiosity has been consistently confused in the psychoanalytic literature in which this battle has been waged. It has been confused with what Kohut called the normal grandiose self. Many of us argued against calling it that because it is always confused with the pathology. But it is not simply a matter of words. There is a vast difference between the configuration Dr. Klein has presented to us, which is pathological and has to be understood as such, and a normal child admiring his father, wanting to be admired by his father as a source of strength for himself or wanting to be admired and mirrored and responded to by a mother who has a gleam in her eye.

I think Dr. Klein reflects that misunderstanding by his slight tinge of sarcasm in response to the patient's grandiose self without making it clear that he is talking about the pathological grandiose self.

Of course, if you were stuck with old psychoanalytic theory, you have nothing to do. That is what Kohut did and wrote about, and that is why he changed his mind. You have nothing to do but say, in effect, "You have to get over this pathological, self-centered, entitled attitude. Look what it's doing to you!"

One of the methods was either subtle or not so subtle disapproval. One of the things that has not been pointed out is that patients all have an enormous need to comply with their therapist. I don't think that need has been sufficiently understood, as to why, in every framework, some things work and the patient goes along with you to a certain extent.

The pathological grandiosity is a consequence of distorted development, insufficient development of the normal, call it the proud, self for the time being. The childhood and adolescent self that is proud, that is expansive, and that has independent initiative as long as it is supported, has the naive, "Look ma, no hands" attitude which is a world apart from pathological grandiosity. The counterpart of the "Look ma, no hands" is the wide-eyed child who is looking up to the parents, admiring them, wanting to be like them, and wanting to lean on, share in, and experience their strength as a source of his or her own strength.

When that is not disrupted, pathologically and chronically, as it was in the first case, some of that feeling of strength and strengthening gets taken in and taken over. That brings us back to the flirtation because that is exactly what the Masterson group wants to do. But they think of the process as different.

The center core of this patient (Mr. Rosen) is relatively better established than that of the first patient, Kate. You don't treat people so differently so much as you understand them differently. It is your understanding of the difference in the core pathology that leads you then to explain something different to the patient, which is what treatment is. You don't say to the man, "You are chronically falling apart because . . ." You wouldn't say this is "because your self-regulatory structures are not intact." But you do say that, in effect, to the first patient.

This man's relatively well established core cohesion, which has been holding together, is threatened all the time, since the breakdown, with severe deflation and desperation. And he is sustained by neither an adequate experience of himself in the pull of the "Look ma, no hands" orginally nor in the pull of relying on strengths of his own that have been internalized. He is literally not struggling to hold together. But he is now deprived within, in the adult personality, of the sustenance that comes from normal mirroring and normal idealizing of a father's strengths and of a mother's strengths.

This normal pull of the proud self is practically not in evidence in Dr. Klein's initial workup. It is atrophied, distorted, barely viable. It is the conscious, loud, noisy organization that has taken the place of the normal idealizing attitude towards the lost father and the normal expectation of building self-esteem through mirroring. What has taken place is that this boy organized or reorganized himself around remnants of the normal proud self. It is called disintegration products by Kohut.

These remnants of a once proud little boy are themselves hypertrophied. He has become the best sufferer, I don't think you have to be sarcastic anymore when you recognize that this is the pathology. What has to grow is the proud, normal self.

He is the best sufferer. He has, as they say in psychoanalytic jargon, sexualized his pain and his suffering and he wants that acknowledged now because there is such a distortion of any kind of expectation or hope of normal mirroring.

The underpinnings of ambitions are inadequate. That is why he can't work. That is why he can't exert himself. There is not sufficient inner structure to take the initiative for sustained and sustaining work. Don't forget that work is sustaining, that is why we do it. We don't just do it because we're good people and adhere to the Protestant ethic, we're sustained by it.

The pathological, inflated self, the Job self, the whatever other self, the cocksman, if you will, bursts all the time like a balloon because it doesn't have any underpinning.

So what is a real depression? This is a real depression, but it is not the depression of old, it is not the depression of middle age. It is the depression of depletion and despair of middle life.

Finally, I am sure the childhood memory of the bums is really fascinating. It's what in self psychology has been called a telescope memory—not a screen memory, a telescope memory. It may refer to the threatening disillusion and disintegration of the father self, to this boy's panic and beginning disorientation, and to the beginning of greater restriction of his development. He had a core of admiring his father, which can be remobilized in his normal development. That is why he became afraid of the bums.

And then Dr. Klein's next sentence is that his father died when the son was 10. So this may be the beginning deterioration and loss of this strengthening father.

Dr. Klein: And that was clearly the sense of it in the treatment. That was the experience for him.

Dr. Masterson: During the course of a normal flirtation, the more experience and interaction we have, the closer the flirtation becomes. I trust that as we move from the borderline to the narcissistic disorder, the flirtation strengthens and turns out to be based more on reality than fantasy, as many flirtations are.

I can't really begin discussing this case without, again, making the point of differential diagnosis. I view the narcissistic disorder's intrapsychic structure as quite different from the borderline personality disorder in the form of intrapsychic structure and in the content. It is this difference in intrapsychic structure which determines the difference in therapeutic technique.

The borderline personality disorder has split self and object representations. The narcissistic disorder has fused self-object representations, which also differ in content, omnipotence and grandiosity, entitlement, and so forth.

I want to discuss differential diagnosis further because I think one of the most confused areas in this field is the diagnosis of the closet narcissistic disorder, the type that Dr. Klein presented. The difficulty springs from the fact that the patient does not come in with an exhibitionist self and also generally isn't able to maintain continuity of his defensive grandiose self, but instead idealizes the object. As a result, the tendency is to look upon him as borderline, like our prior patient, Kate, and then to start doing confrontations. Of course, if that happens, then the treatment fails.

The way you go about establishing a therapeutic alliance with the borderline is through confrontation. The patient's response seems to be based on a sense that, as he internalizes your confrontations, his life, which was chaotic, begins to take some shape and form over which he has some control.

Although the therapeutic objective with a narcissistic disorder is the same, the therapeutic technique differs. The patient is either projecting the omnipotent object upon the therapist, which we call the idealizing transference, or he is exhibiting his grandiose self. You cannot get at this through confrontation. The way we help the patient convert transference acting out into transference and therapeutic alliance is through mirroring interpretation of narcissistic vulnerability.

What happens here in terms of patient experience is quite different than with the borderline. The narcissistic patient begins to form a therapeutic alliance because he feels understood, because he feels that what you are reflecting back to him accurately reflects his intrapsychic experience. We then allow a therapeutic alliance to form, which forms the basis for the work which is basically the analysis of the narcissistic transference.

The window and vehicle for the work has to do with this interpretation . . . interpretation of narcissistic vulnerability. So you can see that we are flirting because we are much closer together here than with the borderline. But I think it's of prime importance, from our perspective at least, to keep clear that the reason for the difference is the difference in diagnosis.

Dr. Sifneos: I tend to view this brief therapy that this particular patient has received as a magnificent result. Many of you have the notion that this is what we're talking about when we talk about short-term psychotherapy. In the sense that we have some transference cure and the patient feels better, we point to what we have done so quickly while others take years.

But this is not the situation here. This particular patient has not been evaluated correctly by his therapist. Once he had been evaluated correctly, he would have seen, of course, all this narcissistic quality in his character structure. Therefore, he shouldn't have been treated by short-term psychotherapy.

But I don't want to give you the impression that people like the ones I'm talking about don't exist. During the coffee break several people were saying that personality disorders, borderline characters, narcissistic personalities, and psychotic people are a product of our society, of our culture. That is why we see more and more of them and psychoneuroses no longer exist. But, of course they exist. They exist by the millions, but they may not come to see you or us or anyone else because we have given the message that we're interested only in very sick individuals and therefore, the ones who have somewhat more circumscribed types of problems continue and lead to divorce and other difficulties we are all familiar with.

Let us be realistic here. We have, in a sense, successful outcomes of these two cases. We shouldn't forget that. We also have, in a sense, no follow-up. We have here some successful results and some follow-up and I want to ask Dr. Tolpin about her follow-ups, or at least the Kohutian approach in terms of follow-up. What research has been done in this particular subject? It's nice to talk about it in great detail and speculate in terms of how many angels can dance on top of a pin. But, finally, results are what count and I'm impressed that we have some meaningful results by this particular approach.

Dr. Tolpin: Approximately 20 years have passed since Kohut came on the scene with a really radically different view, finally getting himself out of libido theory and object relations terms and into English, as some people put it. Our learning this new view has occupied most of us who are clinicians.

The clinicians have follow-ups just like the Masterson group. I would say the Masterson group are extraordinarily open and candid; they don't minimize difficulties. We see some people who are enormously benefitted, who could never have benefitted from earlier psychoanalytic approaches. We see people who are moderately benefitted and we see some people who are not benefitted. Systematic follow-up on this will make possible the next era of clinical advance through our understanding of what is deficient about the outlook, what is an improvement, what is not an improvement. However, only a small group of people, primarily clinicians, are involved in the research efforts and it's going to take time.

But I will say that I am still biased about how fundamentally new insights come. They arise from the psychoanalytic situation, in my view. There has not been any radically new and fundamental insight that's been put to the clinical test that hasn't come out of the psychoanalytic situation and out of the mind of the clinician. I think that is true from Freud to Kohut and all the people in between. That is what we are doing here, and then we talk about the applications. From a scientific standpoint, this approach leaves a lot to be desired. But that's one of the problems in our field.

Dr. Klein: Dr. Masterson, do you feel that, as Dr. Tolpin suggested, we do not give sufficient attention to this distinction between pathological narcissism and normal healthy narcissism?

Dr. Masterson: Obviously, I would deny that. I think that our attention to the healthy narcissism in borderline patients or in narcissistically disordered patients is reflected through the therapeutic alliance, through the support we offer in the therapeutic alliance, through our assumptions and expectations about their capacities to manage, and through our support of what I call real self-activation.

I want to briefly answer the question Dr. Sifneos raised. In my career I have been a researcher and have completed three follow-up studies, which is really more than one human life should have to tolerate. I found out one of the reasons people don't do follow-up studies: They don't want to find out what happened because then all their fantasies of immortality and greatness are dampened.

At any rate, we did research our point of view about treatment of the borderline and it is published in a book called *Borderline Adolescent to Functioning Adult: The Test of Time*. These were borderline adolescents treated in our unit and we did a seven-year follow-up of them as systematically as possible. And we reported all that in this volume.

Question: The mirroring interpretation of Narcissistic Vulnerability has as a primary role defense analysis as a way of not reinforcing the grandiosity. Doing just mirroring without the interpretation may reinforce the grandiosity. In self psychology, are there concerns that if you don't provide that defense analysis you run the risk of reinforcing the narcissistic grandiosity?

Dr. Tolpin: Again we have a problem here because sometimes we use the same terms but mean something quite different. The mirroring interpretation is something that would need to be clarified.

The primary work here would be to do much of what Dr. Klein did, but not with the confrontation of a sit-down strike. The resistance here is shame, the defense against getting more involved for fear of exposing this vulnerable self. Resistance and defense mean the same thing.

In addition, this patient, Mr. Rosen, has the terrible, devastating experience of empty depression that led to his hospitalization. That depression would be regarded as absolutely crucial and the clinical judgement, which actually is demonstrated beautifully here in spite of the theoretical difference, is not to deflate this man while assisting him in the overcoming of the defenses. That was successfully done by a sensitive therapist who has his eye on a normal self, or whatever we call it, that he is addressing.

Again, in terms of this dialogue, the real self that Masterson and his group want to activate and the still existing, normal self that was not totally distorted constitute the object of both groups.

Question: Dr. Tolpin, you alluded to your sense of the differences between the two patients and I wonder if you would expand on that and talk about how that affects your treatment of those patients?

Dr. Tolpin: Well, you know the direction that both cases took, and that's what Dr. Sifneos was referring to, is similar to what the direction might be with the self psychological approach. However, in both cases the concentration on what is going on in the room between you and the patient and that inner experience shows more manifest looking at the patient's "behavior" and less looking at what the patient feels than would be seen in our approach. However, what the patient feels does come out because the defense, the patient's resistance against exposing himself in Dr. Klein's case, is handled so sensitively. The same is true about the other patient, Kate.

But if you attune yourself or put yourself in this man's shoes, which I think Dr. Klein really did, he wouldn't question that he's depressed. I think what you question is calling it a depression and confusing it with other kinds of depression. This kind of depression, though, has been written about by the British Object Relations people. There is a classic paper that I love by one of the British Object Relations people, Enid Balint, called *On Being Empty of Oneself,* which refers to the subjective state of the patient.

Dr. Masterson: I don't think we differ that much in our focus on the inner affective state of the patient, because that's what we're both trying to understand. It may appear on the surface that we differ because of our understanding of the differences in psychological structure between the narcissistic and the borderline. In our view, if you attempted the kind of interventions Dr. Klein made with Mr. Rosen with a borderline patient, you would be reinforcing what we call the rewarding unit and promoting regression.

When we start out with a patient who is defending in behavior, it's not that we're so interested in behavior. Rather, it is the specific defense we must deal with first in order to get a therapeutic alliance and to get in touch with the affectiveness. It is our view that if you go immediately to focus on the inner affective state with a borderline patient, it will lead to regression.

Question: Dr. Tolpin, you have used the word "shame" or you characterized the patient's subjective experience as shame with both patients that were presented. In order to clarify the difference between a self-psychological approach and Dr. Masterson's approach, could you say more about how addressing the issue of the patient's subjective experience of shame is brought into a self-psychological approach? Would it be done differently with a borderline as opposed to a narcissistic patient?

Dr. Tolpin: Again, this question goes back to how you do it. How do you do it with different kinds of patients? And the how you do it comes out of how you understand the basic disorder. You may think you have a patient with a basic disorder, but you could be wrong and you have to keep yourself open to being able to self correct. And how do you do that? You do that with the patient, basically with the patient's reactions to what you're understanding as you communicate it to them.

But what do you do if you have a patient who is chron-

ically in danger of falling apart, not becoming psychotic
but falling apart like this young woman who goes out looking for who knows what and gets raped, or who gorges,
or who uses alcohol? It is your understanding of the patient
that leads you to the interventions that are not the same
as those used with the patient, Mr. Rosen, Dr. Klein talks
about. For example, I would tell the patient Kate that I
know she feels ashamed of herself, that she feels like a
failure as compared to the other people in her family. You
do not have to make these symptoms ego dystonic. You
have to help her with an understanding of why she is so
driven to find the substance. At the same time, you keep
your eye on the beneficial effect of the transference when
it is making for progress: For example, in those early stages
when she was able to accept the idea of going to Alcoholics
Anonymous, she overcame her shame, in other words, and
went to AA. You might tell her she feels too ashamed to
be able to go to Alcoholics Anonymous, but I would not
do so. Dr. Masterson's group would.

Dr. Masterson: Let me respond because you've hit the nail right
on the head, it seems to me. Would you say that, with that
patient who is addicted to alcohol, it would not require
interventions on your part to make the alcoholism ego
alien?

Dr. Tolpin: The alcoholism is manifestly not ego alien. Kate
doesn't come in and say to you, "I can't stand myself because, look, I'm such a mess." That is what she feels. So
you assist her by acknowledging or recognizing that feeling, which is probably a major step that would be useful
in this case.

Dr. Masterson: I disagree with that. I think that what underpins
someone who becomes an alcoholic is the fact that she
sees the symptom behavior as egosyntonic. This is the
defense mechanism of denial and the psychodynamic func-

tion of acting out. The purpose of acting out is to keep yourself from feeling and remembering. So if you take a patient who is an alcoholic, is not feeling, is not remembering, and is denying how destructive the alcoholism is to herself and you say, "I think you feel that you're a mess or you're ashamed about yourself and that's why you drink," I think this comment would fall on absolutely empty ground.

Dr. Tolpin: You know, we may be again talking about the same thing. The purpose of "acting out"—another term I don't like because it's overused and . . .

Dr. Masterson: It is.

Dr. Tolpin: and it's used inaccurately—acting out of the behavior disorder component of the problem is the patient's desire to stay alive, to feel alive, to feel something.

Dr. Masterson: Or not to feel depressed.

Dr. Tolpin: That's right. When the self really is fragmented and there isn't a solid feeling of "I am, I'm real, I can direct myself," you resort to whatever you can in order to make yourself feel alive.

Therefore, you don't have to confront somebody with her denial. You say to her, "You cannot give this up right now because this is how you have organized yourself and made yourself feel alive and what we know is that right now, in this early stage of therapy, you need additional support to deal with it and get yourself off the alcohol while we go ahead with the work." You don't need confrontation.

Dr. Masterson: I think that would be totally useless, literally, with a borderline patient.

Dr. Tolpin: Why?

Dr. Masterson: Because it sounds as if you're reasoning together. With a patient who is so driven to defend against painful affects, you cannot sit down and reason together.

Dr. Tolpin: Well, the patient will say to you, "Yes, that's true," or, "You're full of it," and then you go on and you explore it. Again, I'm not talking about some kind of finished product. This is part of the initiation of the dialogue that doesn't require what you call confrontation, although it does require interventions that involve trying to understand the patient and explaining what you understand to the patient.

Dr. Masterson: In your terms, you are performing a self-object function when you do that. I see this so often in supervision of therapists who are treating borderline patients. The borderline patient is involved, just like this patient, in a whole range of behaviors. I use acting out in a very specific way, which most people don't, as a specific defense against feeling and remembering. When you overcome the acting out through confrontation, without any other interventions needed, the patient starts to feel and remember all those aspects of the depression that they had trouble with in the first place. Too often, therapists try to investigate the depression or the impaired self-cohesion, in the presence of all of this behavioral defense. And what they get is what I call insight as excuse. They get some sort of intellectual compliance that is devoid of the gut-smacking affect the patient has to experience in order to change.

Dr. Tolpin: Well, that's right. You don't sit and say you are ashamed to go to Alcoholics Anonymous.

Dr. Masterson: The patient won't even admit that's necessary, that the alcoholism is a problem.

Dr. Tolpin: You have to take the next step and talk about the shame, in depth, about why the patient experiences it as not necessary and wards it off.

Dr. Masterson: I would never introduce the idea of shame to a patient. I would want the patient to identify that feeling and tell it to me. I think there is such great danger of robbing our patients of their affective states. Freud called the dream the royal road to the unconscious. The affective state is the royal road to acknowledging the self, with all its problems, as a real entity.

Dr. Tolpin: Actually, there is hardly any mention or no mention of shame in the protocol. So, it's an idealistic goal to think that the therapist doesn't take away the patient's initiative. I think that's even a false ideal because there wouldn't be any therapy without the therapist orientation.

There is a great deal of your work that is essentially educational, just as some of it is exhortative and some is highly directive. These are all ways of your mediating self-object functions, as I see it. But nobody conducts theory-less treatment. And so you have to know that the fact that you think about shame and that the patient doesn't even acknowledge it is going to influence what the patient then tells you. Roy Shaeffer said patients will talk Freudian, they'll talk Jungian, they'll talk Adlerian, they'll talk because they need to. And they will even talk Masterson, Sifneos, Kohut, etc. And so it's our job not to fall in love with our theories. That is why we are talking now, because we also have that in common. None of us has so fallen in love with our theories that we are blinded to their limitations and to what the goal is. Otherwise, I don't think I would have been invited. The goal is to improve therapy . . . and I don't come saying that we have the truth in self psychology.

Question: Dr. Tolpin, what I see is a concern about diagnosis and its implications. With Dr. Masterson, we look at diagnosis as important, we try to understand the patient's representation of himself and his object, and we look at the defenses they have and put them into diagnostic configurations without, I think, pretending that everybody is covered. For us it directs the approaches Dr. Masterson has been talking about, whether in terms of what we call confrontation or in interpretation of narcissistic vulnerability. I would ask if you use these types of diagnosis? If not, don't you run the risk of having to have a new diagnosis for every patient?

Dr. Tolpin: Yes, in a sense. There are clusters and, again, that is why we agree. The severe disorder of the self, in my terms, where the center does not hold adequately together and the patient has to enliven herself to try to hold herself together via substances, etc., is your lower-level borderline. So there is a great deal of correspondence. However, from the start we make an effort to make a dynamic formulation. And part of the way you do that is to understand, right from the beginning, how that patient responds to you, how that patient interacts with you, how that patient begins to make use of a certain kind of therapeutic ambience that is established by virtue of your outlook about the patient and how the patient makes use of intervention.

So it's a process that, while it uses everything that you're talking about in terms of the symptom complexes in the configuration, also makes use from the very start of what it is that goes on between you and the patient.

Dr. Masterson: To try to make somewhat explicit what's implicit, it would appear that your focus of observation and emphasis is on the degree of injury to the self and not on a dynamic diagnostic differentiation between borderline and narcissistic. You see the borderline as another version of injured self-cohesion.

Dr. Tolpin: No, Dr. Klein's patient, Mr. Rosen, is an example of a much more holding together center with extreme pathological grandiosity and stunted development in the area of self-esteem and self-sustaining goals. That's the diagnosis.

Dr. Masterson: Okay, that's a self psychology diagnosis. Now, do the same thing for the first patient, Kate.

Dr. Tolpin: I said about the first patient that this is a very severe disorder of self-cohesion. However, she has goals that become possible and she mobilizes goals in the treatment. It emerges that she always had a dream and, therefore, when she goes back for her second Master's, she is now able to sustain herself more with the ambitions and with the goals that she is able to make more solid as a consequence of the treatment. But the primary way of looking at the disorder for diagnostic purposes as a start is that there is really a significant failure in all those realms that make for being adequately able to take yourself for granted sufficiently so that you can get up and do what you have to do.

Question: Dr. Tolpin, I'm still having trouble understanding whether you are talking about a difference in degree or a difference in kind between these two patients?

Dr. Tolpin: We are partly talking about a difference in degree and some of those differences of degree become qualitative differences. Yes, we are talking about a difference in kind.

But first let me say that there is nothing written in self psychology that anybody should quote as gospel. Everything that Kohut said is open to question. As a matter of fact, the great majority of clinicians disagree with what Kohut had to say originally about borderline disorders.

The point that most people would make and that Kohut began to make in the later stages of working with his ideas was that the more you understand your patient, the greater is your access to that person's personality and to what makes him tick, and the more you have a chance to help him. And many of those patients are "less borderline," as you understand them.

Or this may be a consequence of the treatment. Many people who have trouble holding together will, as a consequence of treatment, hold together more with what they have been able to develop. I'm going to give a paper on that at the next self psychology meeting. I'm going to talk about Anna O. I think it's permissible to discuss that here because so much has been mentioned about sexual abuse and about abuse and disassociation. The only thing that hasn't been mentioned is multiple personality.

The story of Anna O. is fascinating because here is a person who was not in good shape. Yet, whatever it is that had happened, she did not have significant disorder in her long, long life from the age of approximately 28 to around 75, when she died. That is the puzzle that self psychology is, in my use of it, at any rate, trying to address. And this is relevant to this borderline issue.

Because your patient may become more sustained, the center may hold and there may be many things that she is able to accomplish in treatment, including getting a Master's Degree in something she really likes. That then becomes self-propelling for her. Does she become less borderline? Or is she just an improved borderline, in your way of thinking about it, by the time she is successfully treated?

Dr. Masterson: In this type of treatment, she will become an improved borderline. That's the objective of the treatment. A borderline who manages.

Dr. Tolpin: So, once a borderline, always a borderline.

Dr. Masterson: No. There may be a little distortion in the first case, that of Kate, because we purposely presented a lower-level borderline first. Later, we are going to present a higher-level borderline. This is a woman of whom I think you are automatically going to say that her center holds together because she is able to function, she does well at work, she is able to function in relationships. In that case, as you work through the abandonment depression, if you're successful, the patient is no longer borderline. She grows out of it.

Dr. Sifneos: Dr. Tolpin, do you consider that the therapeutic results in both of these cases are due to the understanding of their therapists? Or did something else make for these good results?

Dr. Tolpin: The catalytic agent, I believe, is that there is an availability of self-object functions that now can be gradually taken in and taken over. Personalities vary as to how they can do that. I think all of us old-timers, if I may say that, have had the experience of being initially very helpful with patients who do less well than others with whom you wouldn't be as helpful. Haven't you had that experience?

Dr. Masterson: Sure.

Dr. Tolpin: There are mysteries that we have not yet fathomed. There are people who have whole developments we probably don't know anything about. Our histories, our reconstructions, and so forth may really never get to crucial issues that have never been part of whatever people can tell us or that we can fathom. Often, we don't know who is going to get significantly better and who isn't. And it's not directly related to what they are like when they first come to us.

Question: Dr. Tolpin, the two patients described might easily come for help to those of us who work in settings in which we do not have the opportunity to work two, three, four times a week with a patient and where we may be limited to 10 to 20 sessions, whether by time, waiting list, or cost considerations. Do you see in these two patients any focus where you could work with them on a short-term model and still help them in any way? Would you exclude these two patients from any short-term model?

Dr. Sifneos: Absolutely. I would exclude them, absolutely.

Dr. Tolpin: Oh, no. In fact the work really is still incipient in this area. There are enormous applications of the principles of self psychology for brief therapeutic interventions that can have tremendous consequences. For example you can have a consultation with a patient, who is not able to go into treatment with you and you can make an informed recommendation that this patient go to AA, which may have enormous repercussions in the patient's life. You may have to work it out over eight sessions before the patient is able to accept that she should go to AA. That is an example of an intervention in a brief time that would be enormously valuable.

Dr. Sifneos: That's not the kind of brief therapy we are talking about. For instance, seeing somebody briefly to prepare them for analysis is a perfectly legitimate thing, as is getting somebody to go to AA, or accept medications, or whatever.

The kinds of brief therapy we are talking about are, of course, very different.

Dr. Tolpin: There are others, too, though.

Dr. Masterson: I wanted to respond to Dr. Tolpin's answer to Dr. Sifneos. She thinks that what helps patients change is first the therapist's understanding. He has to understand what's going on in all approaches. But then Dr. Tolpin's response was that it probably has to do with a patient's ability to use the self-object functions that the therapist provides. I would rephrase that from our point of view:

It is the patient's capacity to internalize and identify with the therapist's interventions. However, these self-object functions (I'm trying to use both perspectives) have got to be specific to the problem of the patient. Thus, from our point of view, the self-object function with the borderline would be confrontation and with the narcissistic disorder would be these mirroring interpretations. If we reversed it and did mirroring interpretations with a borderline or if we used confrontations with a narcissistic disorder, treatment would go nowhere.

Question: Dr. Tolpin, you say you do see some differences in kind between these two patients, as well as some differences in degree. I confess it still seems a bit amorphous to me here.

Given the fact that you would diagnose these two patients somewhat differently, given the categories that you just described, would they dictate substantial differences in the way you would intervene with these patients? If so, could you briefly characterize the kinds of differences that would be there?

Dr. Tolpin: It's a little late in the morning for me to answer your question as precisely as you would like. But as a rough and ready answer, I would say that the function you offer the patient of grasping his state when you say, "You know, I think you need treatment and you need to go to Alcoholics Anonymous," is just inappropriate to say to Ralph Klein's patient. You wouldn't tell this patient to go to the hospital and have a protected environment, or to join a self help group. The assessment of this patient needs, or what comes out of the assessment, is that he needs an engagement in working with a person to understand the basis of this terrible depression of middle age. In the course of that, you learn about the loss of sustaining inner capacities with the falling apart of his father much earlier than the actual death.

Then you begin to understand what the transference is like. It is not to God, even though he may wish him to be God. Don't we all? This patient is devastated when he senses anything that isn't what he wishes for and needs. And you tell him about that. Dr. Masterson's point is correct. You are off the track if you say to Kate, the young woman patient, "You lost your father's strengths when you were a little girl, you turned to yourself, you hypertrophied all the good qualities that still remained, you made yourself into this suffering godlike creature, and nothing sufficiently sustains you. You can't stand it when I make a mistake or when I go away, or whatever, and you feel again the threat of that inner collapse." That is how you would make a genetic, dynamic formulation to Ralph Klein's patient, Mr. Rosen.

To Kate you say, "You need these strengthening functions." You tell her to go and get them and how to get them and you continuously do that in the therapy.

5

Short-Term Dynamic Psychotherapy

Peter E. Sifneos, M.D.

Short-term interventions are not new. Some of the earliest ones were done by Freud, who treated the case of Dora in nine months.

However, as the analysts became progressively more enthusiastic, they began putting everybody on the couch and moved away from the (Kraepelinian) kind of psychiatry of the 1900s to the psychiatry of DSM-III-R in the 1990s. Many of these patients were psychotic and the analyses were going on and on for long periods of time. Finally in the 20's, two colleagues of Freud, Arthur Rank and Sandor Ferenczi, decided something had to be done to shorten the analysis.

Ferenczi introduced behavior modification techniques in psychoanalysis. They weren't called that at the time, but that's exactly what they were, because he was rewarding and reinforcing his patients in a very interesting way—by somehow telling them the association they had to his confrontation was good. If it was unusually good, he would pat them on the back

Editor's Note: Dr. Sifneos also presented a videotape of an interview with a patient, but we were not permitted to use it. It will, however, be referred to in the discussion.

and tell them it was good. If the association was very, very excellent, he would have them sit on his lap, pat them on the back, and tell them it was good. And if the association was absolutely unique, he would give them a kiss.

As for Arthur Rank, he had a fetish obsession, or whatever you want to call it, about birth trauma, which he viewed as the basic difficulty for all of us. Therefore, the only way to have an analysis, he thought, would be to undo birth trauma by being analyzed only for nine months, since it took nine months for gestation. Well, that was not enthusiastically received and he was asked to leave the International Psychoanalytic Society. We lost these two great attempts to shorten analysis. Freud, himself, wrote a paper and said analysis is terminal and interminable. There are many reasons why some analyses might be interminable: the patient's trauma; very rigid defenses that cannot be broken down; and also the analyst's personality, which may have something to do with that. That's usually pooh-poohed.

Now it was in 1946, after the exodus of analysts from Germany and Austria to North America and Great Britain, that there was an enormous amount of enthusiasm for dynamic processes, which was exciting to see. There was also a demand by the population in general for more and more therapy. In those days there were not enough therapists, so the only way to deal with the demand was through waiting lists. Then a study in London said in 1952 that those who get psychotherapy and those who don't do equally well. Put them on the waiting list and they will be cured.

Well, that was a very infuriating statement. The study also said that there wasn't a single paper that demonstrated effectively the results of psychotherapy or psychoanalysis, because results were mostly on an anecdotal basis.

Franz Alexander and Thomas French wrote a book in 1946 called *Psychoanalytic Psychotherapy*. They talked about manipulating the transference almost in an acting way. Of course, that book was taboo, at least in the Boston Psychoanalytic Society where I was a candidate in training at the time.

Our major industry in Boston is education, and we have a lot of students. Faced with the issue of running a very large psychiatric clinic, we decided to try to do a more systematic evaluation and not simply place them on the waiting list in the hope that somebody would get to see them two or three times a week.

In 1956, an interesting man came in complaining of an acute onset of phobias for all forms of transportation. When he announced his plans to get married in three months, he was evaluated by one of the teams and was told what was classic at the time—that he had a phobic neurosis of acute onset and needed twice-a-week psychotherapy for a couple of years. Don't forget, 1956 was before psychopharmacology and before we had behavior modification for phobias. And he said, "No, I want to get married. I mean, I'm not that sick, but I have this foolish fear." He couldn't get inside a car, a train, a bus, or any vehicle.

He came to see me, since I was the director of the clinic, and I agreed that that was the treatment. He said, "No! Somebody must help me. Would you help me?" I said, "Me? Well, it's not going to work, but let's try."

He had eight interviews and, indeed, his phobias had practically diminished. He was a little bit apprehensive, but he could get inside a car. He was afraid, also, of walking down the aisle on his church ceremony. However, he was optimistic and was looking forward to it.

I told him to come back and see me after the honeymoon. I thought to myself that in all probability, all the symptoms were going to come back. It was kind of a transference cure, but no good at all.

He did come back. He had gone to New York for the honeymoon and he had a great time riding in the subways. He said, "I was terrified, I would have been terrified with these trains,

but I was having a great time." I said, "Come to our Grand
Rounds." People thought you needed two years twice a week,
but we were able to do that in three months time.

He came to Grand Rounds and was interviewed by Dr. Harry
Lindemann, whom some of you may know as the father of
community mental health. I noticed that there were several
members of the Boston Psychoanalytic Society, where I happened to be a candidate-in-training at the time, who were invariably frowning. As soon as the patient left, one got up and
said that what I had thought was a transference cure was no
good. Another one said it was a flight into health. No good!
Another one said it might be a counterphobic response. No
good! I pointed out that the patient seemed to be happy. That
didn't make any difference at all. One came up to me and said,
"Sifneos, you're a candidate at the Institute, are you not?" I
said I was. He said, "You want to graduate, don't you?" I said
I did. He said, "Don't you know what happened to Ferenczi?"
I thought he was joking. He continued, "Who ever heard of
short term? Don't you know it takes a long time for the human
mind to change?"

In a state of panic and anger, I went straight to my supervisor.
I was lucky enough to have a superb supervisor, Dr. Elizabeth
Zetzel. She said what I had to do was find out about the parameters of the patient's character structure. What she was
telling me was to find other people with similar types of character structure and try to treat them in this short-term way. I
asked how I could find 10 or 15 people who were going to get
married in three months time and had developed phobias of
all forms of transportation. "Of course not," she said, "just find
out what were the parameters of the character structure." What
she meant was "criteria for selection."

What were they? First, acute onset of a circumscribed symptom, the phobias. Otherwise, functioning perfectly well. Second, good, adequate, give-and-take interactions. I can go into
great details for that, but it is what we call a meaningful relationship, a give-and-take relationship with one person during

early childhood. Therefore, this is not the chaotic type of experiences characterizing the cases, for instance, that were presented today or others you undoubtedly know only too
well.

Third, ability to interact meaningfully with the evaluator. Not
only was he able to interact with me, but he convinced me to
do something which I was against and we were able to have a
successful outcome.

Fourth, he was psychologically minded. Fifth, he was facing
a crisis—namely, three months time to get married. And, sixth,
he was motivated to change. He said repeatedly, "I know that
these things come from me. I'll do anything I can if I find
someone to help me resolve this particular problem."

With these six criteria for selection, in the next four years
we found 50 patients, 21 of whom we saw in a follow-up of
two years. Now 50 patients in four years is a ridiculously small
number and some people here were saying during coffee break
that, of course, these patients don't exist. Even Jim Masterson
told me they don't exist—at least in New York.

But, nevertheless, we decided to look at those patients in
follow-up two years later. The main thing they said was, "I
learned a great deal about myself and I can now overcome by
myself some of the problems I was facing in the past." When
I heard the word "learning," we attributed this as a cognitive
change. We didn't pay any attention to it. The fact was that it
was there. Self-esteem greatly improved. Relationships with
other people greatly improved.

We were encouraged so we presented those 21 patients at
the American Psychiatric Association's annual meeting. I was
told that Franz Alexander was going to be my discussor. Well,
he and French had written that book, *Psychoanalytic Psychotherapy*, which I knew nothing about. Imagine your discussor
asking what you think of his book and you have never heard
of it. Also, the day before the presentation, *The New York
Times Magazine* had a picture of Franz Alexander and a big
write-up about him. He was quoted as saying that when dis-

cussing papers he disliked he had a tendency to tear the presenter apart.

So with this very reassuring situation, I presented my paper the next day. The place was jammed, of course, for Franz Alexander. After my presentation, he said in this heavy Hungarian accent, "Criteria for selection of 50 patients, my God, when there are millions of people who could benefit from this approach. For heaven's sake, go back to Boston, loosen up the criteria for selection, and you'll see many more patients."

Well, which criteria should we give up, considering that we thought they were all important? One was the acute onset of symptoms. People who had acute onset of symptoms went to the emergency floor of the hospital. Therefore, they were not coming to the psychiatric clinic. So we dropped the acuteness.

Then there was the crisis situation. Here, too, patients would go to the emergency floor, which was under the direction of an entirely different group of people from our department.

Having dropped the crises and the acuteness, within the next four years we got more than 500 patients. So the patients were there. We hadn't seen them because we were so rigid in our approach to selecting.

We got excited about that and we went to London to the international Congress where I met Dr. David Malin. He said that in England they called what we were doing "brief psychotherapy." He also said we have to once and for all knock out the statement of Isaacs that patients did as well without psychotherapy. He said we know that some people get well with psychotherapy and some don't, but it is important to demonstrate results adequately through controlled research studies.

And that's what we did. It was much easier to do it in Boston rather than in England where they have the National Health Service and the general practitioners act as a filter. Instead of sending these people to specialists like a psychiatrist, they keep them and they pat them on the back or give them a pill.

We asked two independent evaluators to assess the patients without communicating with each other and then to specify in writing what criteria for outcome would satisfy them that the patients' problems had been resolved. The prospective patients were matched according to age and sex. Those taken immediately into therapy were the experimental ones; the controls waited without therapy until the end of the treatment of the experimental patients. The treatment, usually once a week, face to face, lasted three to six months.

Then the untreated control patients were called back. What changes had taken place during the waiting period without benefit of psychotherapy? If the London study were correct, both groups would have done essentially the same. Well, they hadn't. Sometimes some of these control patients had symptomatic improvement. However, in terms of criteria for outcome, which are vital and are what the evaluators had to write down, there was nothing that would satisfy a dynamically oriented person that indeed the patient had enough insight, nor could any recovery be attributed to this insight.

On the other hand, we had very adequate findings for the experimental group who were treated right away. When the control patients then were given the same type of therapy, they had exactly the same findings as the experimental ones.

As I said, we had only 30% of a follow-up. The difficulty in this huge country, particularly with a lot of students, is to try to get them back three or four years later. That is why I went to Norway where I presented these same findings. They shook their heads and said these people might exist in America, but not in Norway. I said that they do exist in Norway, but the therapists haven't been looking for them.

Well, not only did we find them, but we trained the therapists in how to treat them and how to use video, which was vital. They had a five-year follow-up, which was much better than ours since they covered 90% of the patients, with exactly the same findings as we had. The control patients did not change without benefit of therapy, but after they were treated in the same way as the experimental patients, they, too, changed dramatically.

We don't have time here to go into describing the techniques, which are dynamically oriented, but quite different. We use the transference immediately, as soon as it appears. We don't wait for it to appear as a resistance. We're anxiety-provoking. Knowing that the patients have solid character structures, but with a deficiency in this one circumscribed area, we can push them and we can push them hard. We establish what we call past/present linking—that is, links of experiences they had with key people in the past, which are now transferred under therapy to bring them alive during the therapeutic interaction. We are active. We don't put them on our lap and give them a kiss. We are active in order to keep the patient on the focus. Focality, of course, is a vital issue.

There is tangible evidence of change when the therapist can see that the patient is utilizing different defense mechanisms, much more adaptively, in the area of the problem that has been selected as the focus. Most of these problems are grief reactions, loss or separation, or unresolved oedipal problems. Then, it is time to terminate. It is interesting that at least 50% of our patients introduced the thought that it was time to terminate because they were behaving in a very different way. And if you agree with them, of course it's adequate. You have to make sure that they're not acting out.

We did six studies like this, trying more and more to have as homogeneous a group of people as possible. In the last two studies, we have picked up patients who had unresolved oedipal problems, according to the criteria that I mentioned to you, and this was the focus of the therapy.

By the late 60s we got what I call the microscope, which is essentially the ability to show what the patients look like at the time of the evaluation. You can show each and every interview of the therapy and then, most important, see the long-term follow-up. That long-term follow-up is the proof of the pudding.

We have always been criticized. I remember many faculty meetings at Harvard Medical School when someone—the neurologist, particularly—would get up and say, "Of course, psychiatry is a pseudo science," and he would have that supercilious smile on his face, because we had nothing to demonstrate.

6

Discussion of Short-Term Dynamic Psychotherapy

Question: Is the therapist always active?

Dr. Sifneos: The activity of the therapist is crucial. We don't have time and we don't want to have a transference neurosis on our hands when we can't use free association to analyze it, and so forth. But in all our tapes, you can see that we are active. We are not active in Ferenzczi's terms, but we are active in terms of staying on the focus.

The focus of the patient discussed was her relationship with her father, which reflected in her relationships with men and her husband. Actually, her husband was an American who studied in Spain and then came to New York. And she had not passed the bar exam, even though she had a law degree from Barcelona, and one year in London. She wants to divorce her husband, who loves her, and wants to go back to the hornet's nest in Spain to be with that sadistic father who treats her one way and then treats her in another way, like a lover.

Question: I was concerned about your saying that she had a good relationship with her father. It seems to me, diagnostically, that the mother was borderline and the father narcissistic. She was taking care of the mother and the father did not love her. He was sexually interested in her, but he did not love her. And you kept saying that he loved her. I don't see that she had a good relationship with either parent. She did seem to have a good relationship with her grandmother.

Dr. Sifneos: The relationship with her grandmother is the key. You see, we want to have one meaningful, give-and-take relationship with somebody in childhood. She had five years with that grandmother, who was actually like a mother to her.

The second thing is that as bleak as she presents her relationship with her father, still she interacts very well with me. So, obviously, there is something in that relationship with her father that involved a conflict. On the one hand she was attracted to him and he was attracted to her. At the same time he treated her in a very bad way. That was one of the aspects of the conflict.

But how did she relate to her husband? How did she relate to all these other men, including me in the evaluation interview? Obviously, she had learned it from somewhere and I think she learned it from that skewed relationship with her father.

Question: I have to confess a bit of skepticism in that, I'm always tempted, if I have to present a tape, to present one that fits my views. It seemed to me that you were focusing on oedipal issues right away and very selectively identifying them. This approach seemed to fit this patient's particular problem. Is that typical of the patients you work with? Do you usually get this corroborating evidence of oedipal issues if you look at the patients in this fairly single-minded way?

Dr. Sifneos: Absolutely. At that time when I saw this lady in New York, although she was not part of our research group, we were having a research study whose focus was the unresolved oedipal problem with these patients who fulfill the criteria for selection, as you have seen in this particular lady.

As I said, I knew nothing about this patient in the beginning. However, the information she was giving me reminded me of a great number of patients whom we see in Boston.

So I'm not showing you carefully selected successes. This is a research project and there's a whole library of video tapes of these particular patients. You can see them if you come to Boston.

Question: Well I'm curious in terms of style and what happens in this treatment process. What kind of affect emerges?

Dr. Sifneos: One of the things that we pick up immediately and observe very carefully is any transference feeling a patient may have for the therapist. Invariably, we see that the positive feelings predominate. Essentially, there are these people who have the capability of expressing positive feelings for someone. In that sense, they are not these sicker patients who are the subject of this symposium. This is a significant differential.

The second thing is the motivation. We heard what a difficult time the cases that were presented here were giving to their therapist because their motivation was dwindling or went through peaks and valleys. The people we treat work very hard and very quickly.

So the selection of the appropriate patients, plus working on the focus, which we agree upon at the time of the evaluation, and using the special technical devices is what we feel is responsible for the improvement in these particular patients seen in the follow-up. These factors also help assure the adequate follow up we have for many studies.

I don't want to go into all the details of what the patients tell us, but one of the things that they tell us most clearly is that they can utilize what they have learned from this experience in therapy in solving new problems in their lives. Therefore, they don't need to have a therapist to go to for further treatment. In a sense, this therapy becomes a preventive tool against future difficulties.

Question: You said you were focusing for a variety of reasons on oedipal issues. In our reading about character pathology in general, we looked closely at pre-oedipal issues, separation, and abandonment. Do you focus on those things briefly? Do you, in some cases, look in that direction instead?

Dr. Sifneos: No. We are not going to focus on them. Although they might exist, they exist, I think, as they do in all of us. We all have gone through some of those phases, but they are not as intense and overwhelming as they are with these sicker patients. Therefore, we concentrate on the unresolved oedipal problem. We concentrate, for instance, on unresolved grief reactions and on loss and separation issues; we don't have the major, catastrophic, regressive-like ways which we have seen in the much sicker patients presented here. That is why we can keep the situation on a much more short-term basis in this very active way of staying within a particular focus.

I think everybody who has done this work agrees on that point. Here in San Francisco, as a matter of fact, Dr. Marge Hall's group at Langley Porter have emphasized the loss and separation issue, and have done very systematic work on that area of the focus. This is the difference. You cannot go on everything.

On the other hand, if you select patients who have major

difficulties in their pre-genital character structure, obviously you cannot do this kind of work.

Question: I would be curious to have you speak directly to how
you make a differential. You obviously gather a lot of
information actively. Are there patient responses that
would tell you that the patient is a character disorder and
not suitable for your work?

Dr. Sifneos: Yes. Actually, that is a very important point in
terms of your going over the criteria for selection and
finding out that indeed there wasn't anybody in the relationship as a child.

Another of the criteria involves how the patient interacts
with you, the evaluator. You must decide how the patient
relates. For example, if the patient relates very well, is
open and tells me that she is angry with me, I then have
an opportunity to see if I can make a past/present link
interpretation.

Dr. Masterson: I would like to underline how beautifully Dr.
Sifneos' approach illustrates the difference between personality disorders and people who have higher level arrest
at the oedipal level.

There are a number of things that he can take for
granted. For example, he does not have to help the patient
convert transference acting-out into therapeutic alliance
and transference. He starts out assuming a transference
exists. The reason we can't link past with present at the
beginning of treatment is that the patient is unable to do
it because of the transference acting-out. Dr. Sifneos can
do it right in the first session and the patient picks it up.

Thus, we have him starting out at a point which is an
achievement for us in psychotherapy. It takes a lot of time
and it is an achievement for us to achieve a secure therapeutic alliance. He starts out with the assumption that he

has it and that gives him a great deal of latitude with his interventions.

I would be curious to ask him: Other than history, what kinds of things would you see going on in the session that would make you begin to wonder and back off and maybe explore that the patient was a character disorder?

Dr. Sifneos: Well, I think it would come back to the interaction with the evaluator. I think that would probably be the acid test.

Dr. Masterson: What would you expect to see? What kinds of things might happen?

Dr. Sifneos: For instance, when I would challenge a patient's notion of her positive relationship with her father, she might become angry at me and continue being angry at me.

Dr. Masterson: In other words, you are saying that she was involved in a projection which did not yield to the reality relationship with the therapist; therefore, there was not a sufficient therapeutic alliance.

Dr. Sifneos: Yes.

Dr. Tolpin: I would like to ask some questions. Would you comment on two things? What do you think has taken place as a result of making somebody conscious in this very focal way of something of which they had been previously unconscious? And what do you think of the labors over many years of those who have worked at psychoanalysis and thought that an unconscious oedipal conflict was responsible for a great many problems in the personality, not excluding the group that turns out not to have an oedipal conflict central at center? Yet, all kinds of inhibitions, symptoms, anxiety, and so forth were attributed to an oedipal problem. What do you think about the analytic work that continues to focus in long-term analysis on such problems, regards them as crucial, and requiring a long-term working-through process?

Dr. Sifneos: Well, in terms of the first question, I don't think that this lady's oedipal problem was unconscious. I think she was quite aware. I mean there might be a preconscious, or even conscious, awareness of these particular problems. And it wasn't something which might have been much more difficult to get out into the open.

In terms of the second question about how the analyst continued to go on, I think this is his or her problem and not the patient's.

7

Intensive Analytic Psychotherapy of a Borderline Personality Disorder

Karla R. Clark, Ph.D.

CASE PRESENTATION

My patient is 45 years old. She is a practicing attorney who presently lives alone. She has been in psychotherapy for six years. For the first year and a half, she saw me first once and then twice a week. About 18 months into treatment, she began to come three times a week and to use the couch.

In a therapy this long, there is an enormous amount of material to discuss. For my purposes today, I have chosen to trace one particular strand of the treatment—the management of the patient's use of the defenses of detachment of affect and compliance at the beginning of therapy and late in the working-through period.

Presenting Complaint

The patient, whom I will call Mrs. A, asked for help with a pervasive low-level feeling of depression which she claimed to have experienced throughout most of her life. Her live-in arrangement with her lover of seven years, Mr. B, was in bad shape. The couple quarreled frequently about money, life-style, and degree of commitment (she wanted marriage, he was adamantly opposed to it). They drank too much and had a poor sex life. Despite the fact that he manifestly had many problems, they had a consensus that the problem was mostly because of the *patient's* depression. As an illustration of her compliance and clinging, she agreed with him that if she could "fix" that depression, their relationship would be satisfactory.

Treatment History

Mrs. A had first sought treatment for depression during college. She remembers nothing about this experience except that it was brief and unsatisfactory. She had once again turned to psychotherapy, some 10 years later, under circumstances similar to those which eventually brought her to me: Her first marriage was going badly and she was experiencing depression. She saw a psychologist for five years, once and sometimes twice a week. From her reports, she had evidently clung to the therapist. She divorced during this period, had several affairs, and then became involved with her current lover, Mr. B. Her therapy ended abruptly when her therapist stood up one day while she was in the middle of a sentence and left the room, offering no explanation. The patient said nothing to him when he returned. She reports having experienced no feelings whatsoever, but she left the session at its end and never went back. At the time when she consulted me, some three years later, she had difficulty in remembering the therapist's name. Her report of her handling of this incident was the first evidence I had of her detaching defense.

Patient's History

The patient is the oldest of three children. Her parents are divorced now, but did not separate until the patient was an adult.

During the Second World War, her father was in the service. The patient and her mother lived with her maternal grandparents. The patient reports a very positive and affectionate relationship with her grandmother during this important time in her life.

The father returned from the service when the patient was three and the family moved some distance away from the grandparents' home. Mrs. A say them infrequently after that.

The parents' marriage was extremely tense. The father was an alcoholic, a womanizer, and prone to violent rages. The mother was passive, insensitive, and emotionally remote.

The father was physically very violent with all three of the children. He also sexually molested the patient when she was seven years old by crawling into her bed and fondling her genitals. She recalls pretending to be asleep and praying for the experience to be over. She never told anybody about this, although she never forgot the incident. Though he never actually molested her again, during the rest of her years at home her father was sexually inappropriate. Detaching, she spoke to me of these experiences with no feeling.

Her mother, who witnessed many of the incidents involving Mrs. A and her father, appeared unaware and never interfered on her daughter's behalf. In counterpoint to the unprotective attitude which the mother had toward her daughter in these situations, in others the mother was prone to take over and do things for the patient which she was able to do for herself. Mrs. A experienced her mother, for the most part, as both her protector and somebody whom she needed to protect. She rarely criticized her mother. At the start of treatment, Mrs. A described her relationship with her mother as "symbolic," by which she meant poorly differentiated. They cared for one another and neither experienced the other as a truly separate entity.

Despite the tension and difficulties at home, Mrs. A did well in school and also was able to establish many friendships. As she grew older, she tried to spend as little time at home as possible, preferring to visit in the homes of her friends. During high school, she also met and began to date her first husband over the objections of his more socially prominent family.

After graduating from high school, the patient continued school while living at home. The parents' opposition to and attacks on her attempts at education intensified. After a particularly violent fight, she packed and fled with the help of her boyfriend. She got a small apartment of her own and a job. Clinging, she married her boyfriend immediately upon graduating rather than accepting a scholarship for graduate work.

Detaching, almost from the start the patient felt unemotional toward her husband and, clinging, began to have affairs outside of her marriage.

She also managed to leave her husband by having an affair (clinging) and detaching affect (she never consciously mourned the relationship). She moved in with his replacement, lived with him briefly, and then had a series of other affairs, culminating in her meeting and living with Mr. B. During this time, she did decide to go to law school. She managed to graduate, neither at the top nor bottom of her class, and passed the bar on the second attempt.

Diagnosis

This history reveals major difficulties in managing those aspects of the self which have to do with psychological separation, mainly in the establishment and maintenance of intimacy.

The patient also had difficulty with individuation in that her interests, while diversified and identifiable, were never really crystallized nor were her really formidable talents fully channeled.

Her major defenses were splitting, detachment of affect, clinging, acting out the wish for reunion, denial, and intellectualization. There was clear evidence of the borderline triad, in which efforts she made in her own behalf were quickly followed by evidence of both depression and defenses.

I diagnosed the patient as a moderately high-level borderline.

Course of Treatment

Her tendency to cling through compliance was rapidly mobilized in the treatment in the form of being a "good" patient, rarely late, paying her bills on time, always polite, never angry at me, eager to listen to what I had to say and to use it.

While this compliance has its own set of problems, I was more concerned, from the point of view of prognosis, about the way that she had detached affect in order to manage her feelings around the termination of her last attempt at therapy. In fact, I discovered as I began to work with her that she lived most of her life in that detached state. She was like a sleep-walker most of the time, wandering around the edges of life, rarely feeling, rarely experiencing what happened to her.

Therapy began once a week. The patient immediately demonstrated both sides of her conflict: She tried to be a "good patient" and please me on the one hand and was detached and intellectualized on the other. When confronted, she would contain the detachment and cling, contain the clinging and detach. Here is an example of how this was handled. In the third session, she told me that she was concentrating on relaxing as a way to deal with feelings of anxiety. Addressing her detachment, I asked her why she chose to focus on that rather than on trying to understand her anxiety. She replied, revealing the clinging component of her behavior, "I'm bringing here what I do in my practice. I have done it all of my life. I feel a pressure to succeed, to be liked, to be a good client. I am doing it right now, thinking of saying the right thing." I asked her how she felt and she said, crying, "I feel blocked, caged, like, whatever you do is not going to be right. I feel crazy, I do. At least I limit it to here. I'm sitting here groping for things to talk about, censoring myself, trying to be a good girl without knowing the rules. Like when I was a little girl. Different things were expected. My mother—there were times when she wanted to be close to me and times she didn't. She would generate fights between me and Dad. She'd be on my side and then switch and it was real confusing. I felt abandoned. I guess I never dealt with it. I left home. I avoided them for months."

Toward the end of the session, she said, "I see where situations which I create alienate me from other people . . . (at the same time) I am scurrying around in some frantic manner, trying to please a lot of people I don't trust . . . trying to please somebody I don't trust and on some bottom level I don't care if they like me or I can please them. I think I anticipate in my mind rejection, and that's why I don't get involved. Here, I ask myself, 'Does she like me?' and I say it doesn't matter, it's her job. But that's a defense against rejection. . . . Where to *be* is to consider myself likable, so it doesn't matter so much."

The patient began to experience detachment, in particular, as against her best interests and to begin to try to control it. In the next session, she said, "I am presently not in touch with anything remotely resembling a feeling. I think I should concentrate on my feelings about my mother and how she treated me. It seems real central. But it seems artificial. I guess because I don't want to look at it." Following this, the patient began to speak with feeling about her life with her mother, whom she revealed to be both destructive and pathologically self-protective in her transactions with family members. In this session, work of this sort alternated with periods where she cut off feeling and periods where she tried to be a "good little girl" and give me what she supposed that I wanted. Simply asking her about this was enough at this time for her to stay on track. At the end of the session, she said, "Part of me feels like feeling and part of me says I don't wanna, I'm not gonna do it. And it is frustrating. The feeling, it disengages or something."

The patient went home for the Christmas holidays. Still dealing with her tendency toward detachment, which was seeming more and more distasteful to her, she said, "I am torn between warring factions. The only way to do that is to act like a zombie, and who wants that for yourself? Everybody there lies. I should be honest. I should draw limits. I should get angry, I suppose." She lapsed into compliance. I pointed this out, and she said, "That eagerness to please is a buffer, a screen, so I don't have to look at what an outsider I feel like. So to go to take care of myself makes me see reality, which I don't want to see. . . . There's a big part of me that never gets involved in things at all. That eager to please thing is a mask—most specifically to myself. I feel like a robot. I have an image of the desert—a lot of wind and nothing there. . . . I don't like this. I suppose I have to look at my feelings of loneliness, which are real scarey. I don't like those feelings."

By the end of the third month of treatment, the patient was able to steadily notice her feelings of detachment and was attempting to grapple with them more consistently. "I really feel strange. I feel like I'm not here. All day, a real going through the motions. My head's like a tape machine. I can't think of the right word, and the tape's this self-depreciating one—and, if it stops, there is nothing . . . like there is this void—there's not much point in talking about it."

In the following sessions, her sense of depression deepened. As before, she tried to control it, when not detaching, by clinging. She said, "I get in touch with what I feel. It is kind of feeling, like, abandoned. Yeah. That's how it feels. We talked about feeling in a desert, sort of like there, abandoned, not knowing what you're doing, with no sense of direction. It is because I am afraid to trust you. I'm afraid you won't point me in the right direction." I said, "You begin to take care of yourself trying to identify your feelings and then you turn around and say that you're afraid that *I* won't point you in the right direction?" She said, "It's my laziness. You do it. I want to be adopted. Rather than give up, I've decided I want to be a little kid and have another go at it or something like that. I guess that feeling of being alone is real scary for me."

At this point, four months after her first contact with me, the patient was consistently tracking and overcoming her tendency to detach and coming to understand her clinging helpless behavior as destructive and unnecessary. She was, therefore, less removed in her personal life. For the first time, she began to bring in material which suggested the degree of disturbance in her relationship with her lover, Mr. B. The conflict with Mr. B intensified when she saw more and more clearly his arrogant and depreciating treatment of her. She came to understand that a great deal of what she knew as depression was really a reaction to having consistently allowed Mr. B to take advantage of her. As she stood up to him, the relationship deteriorated.

She found a good job at this point and, with that financial security behind her, left Mr. B. I thought that, at this point, the patient was truly poised to work through.

Under this severe abandonment stress, however, the patient defended. She detached affect, feeling very little anger, grief, emptiness, loss, whatever. Within a week of leaving Mr. B, she clung, by beginning a relationship with Mr. C. He was extremely helpful to her during a severe physical illness. Completely ignoring many warning signs about the degree and kind of Mr. C's own personal problems, she saw him as her white knight. The two quickly became engaged. Since efforts I made to vigorously confront the destructiveness of such a leap from one relationship into another were completely stonewalled by the patient, I turned to pointing out the destructiveness of the patient's clinging *behavior* to her feelings about herself. I hoped that, as she controlled the clinging, she would see the problems in her relationship more clearly. She, however, simply reversed the field: She became strong and maternal, and Mr. C began to cling to her rather than the other way around. She remained unable to see the destructiveness of the relationship and married Mr. C.

With all of this acting out going on, I had grave doubts about the future of the patient's analysis. Interestingly enough, although it was definitely a factor, the bleeding off of affect by acting out was not really apparent for more than three years. In the meantime, she began to make great steps toward improving her functioning at work. She tolerated more and more depression, as memories of early childhood emerged and she began to understand the degree to which she had felt alienated and coopted by her mother. She asserted herself more consistently everywhere in her life except with her husband and began to remake her relationships with her family in a pattern which suited her better.

Her real self was emerging. She went to a family gathering, where she once more confronted her mother's lack of interest and investment in her and her needs. Crying, she said, "I became aware that they wouldn't go with me (to a beloved aunt's grave). I knew that I had to get away by myself for a little while in order to deal with how this made me feel, so that I would not distract myself. I took a walk. The most awful feeling came over me. I can't describe it to you. It was as bad as I have ever felt. And then the most amazing thing happened. Although I continued to feel just terrible, I looked down at the ground and realized that I was walking through the most beautiful leaves. They had such wonderful colors. I reached down and picked them up, and as I walked, I arranged a bouquet. I touched the leaves. I knew again, you see, that my mother would never acknowledge me, not ever. No matter how many times I have told you that I know this, I think that I have never quite given up hope. This time, I think it really sunk in. As bad as I felt, I realized that, somehow, I could mother myself. It's not quite the same. I don't mean that it wouldn't be nice to have a mother and aunts who would go with me to the grave to share those experiences. That's not what I mean. It would be. It would. But it is that, if that is not there, I know now that I have something within myself which can make it o.k. . . . I brought the leaves home on the plane. The leaves have faded now, but it doesn't matter. I can't explain it, but the leaves are inside."

She was now prepared to confront her relationship with Mr. C. She came home full of righteous indignation at a brother-in-law for being so "irresponsible" as to come home two hours late without telling his wife where he was, loudly praising Mr. C, who would never think of doing such a thing. I said, "Mrs. A, which would you rather have—a husband who comes home a couple of hours late without calling or a husband who fails to make mortgage payments consistently, over and over again, jeopardizing your home? A husband who is always drunk? A husband who neglects his physical health in dangerous ways?" She thought and, then, soberly and tearfully answered, "The real answer, of course, is neither. But I see what you mean." Her denial was decisively overcome at this point. She and Mr. C entered marriage counseling, where the marriage counselor confronted her over and over again with the destructive realities of their marriage. She decided to divorce Mr. C.

This time, she experienced the feelings around the separation fully. The barrier to full working through presented by her marriage was decisively breached. There was a marked and dramatic intensification of all of her affects at this juncture, including, for the first time, severe feelings of panic associated with experiencing herself as a separate person. This led to a powerful surge of memory and affect concerning her father's molestation and abusive behavior. She said, "In the beginning, I started out with bad patterns of merging with my mother. I think that is what I thought would protect me from my Dad. Whenever I start thinking about unmerging, I get frightened."

Repeatedly, as this material emerged, she has returned to detachment as a defense against the rage and hopelessness which these experiences of abuse and objectification have generated.

"It wasn't just my dad. It was my mother, too. I know how it worked. He built on, he preyed on, a preexisting condition. I already felt responsible for mother. So it was easy for me to think I was responsible for him as well." She then detached. I reminded her that recently she had said to me that it felt worse to admit to herself that she was not responsible than to retain the feeling of responsibility and, with it, the feeling that she counted. I said that once again it seemed that she was backing away from that feeling. Interpreting, I said, "The feeling is so unbearable that you do things to it. . . . You cut off, or treat yourself like an object, or blame yourself, or accuse me of treating you like an object, all to protect yourself from the awfulness of these feelings."

She replied, "It's true. The feeling is that there is nobody to protect me but me. The world is only there to criticize me. The world is not there to help me out. I was wondering why I try so hard to get people's approval . . . because that doesn't fit with what I have been saying. It is not approval, it is some recognition that I am not an object. I wanted people to think I was a nice person. The operative word here is *person*."

At this writing, this is leading the patient in two directions. One is deeper into anger and hopelessness associated with specific memories of molestation. The other is into a deeper and more involved appreciation of life. Recently, she was trying to evaluate her experience that things are changing greatly inside of her. I will end with her words. "I don't feel as empty as I used to. I am not filled up with people or relationships, but I am filled up more and more with my thoughts and ideas. I am not so empty anymore . . . and that makes a big difference."

8

*Discussion of Intensive
Analytic Psychotherapy of a
Borderline Personality Disorder*

Dr. Sifneos: This is a beautiful psychotherapy of long duration in comparison to what I have just presented and I think it demonstrates so nicely the different kind of people we are dealing with. In this situation, I was looking at the criteria for this particular patient and noted that she had poor relationships with people all along. This is certainly exemplified by the horrendous experience she had with her father, who obviously pulled the rug from under her, which led to the anger that has emerged very recently.

Then there is her relationship with her mother, which is not a relationship at all. Her mother is supposed to protect her and she doesn't protect her at all. There is vaguely a grandmother, but we don't know about her. Certainly, she doesn't fulfill the second of the criteria that I emphasized in my presentation. I'm not clear as to her relationship with you, Dr. Clark, but it is definitely ambivalent, to put it mildly. It isn't a relationship like the positive, working together therapeutic alliance we develop with my patient within the first evaluation interview. Here it takes a long period of time to evolve.

She is obviously an intelligent person and seems to be psychologically minded, so she passes that criterion. But I'm not absolutely certain, about her motivation for change, at least not until she herself feels certain there is a possibility of emerging.

Obviously, we have a wide gamut of psychopathology to deal with here and our interventions vary entirely. That's about all I can say. Certainly, a patient like her would not be a good candidate for short-term dynamic psychotherapy. She needs very long interaction with somebody who is very sensitive, who supports her during that splitting and detachment, telling her she is a good girl, all those things you have emphasized so much.

Dr. Tolpin: I think one of the wonderful things about your case presentation is that it illustrates an attitude you have of expectations of growth. Also, you are not presenting things cut and dried. They're difficult, and you don't minimize the difficulties and you don't hesitate to bring them out.

It is in that spirit that I would comment on some of the differences in the self psychological outlook. In sum, your interventions first aim at, or they foster, ego dominance in autonomy. They don't say, "Pull yourself together." They say, "Get a hold of yourself, look at it, and see what you can do about making a therapeutic split, which is different from the splitting defense."

The aim in self psychology from the very beginning of the treatment is to foster whatever is going to lead to a manageable transference where the understanding of the transference will lead to some internalization and reorganization. Here I'd mark an actual example of an interpretation that I think we could discuss and that would be different from a self psychological point of view, but first let me give you an overview of this case in diagnostical terms.

This is a patient who has had a long-time depletion

depression, an empty depression that she has tried to deal with by filling in through clinging relationships to men. These relationships become like a life raft to her, even though they're abusive, repeating aspects of her relationship with her father. She clings to them. There is no appreciation of her own capacities, which obviously are really significant.

Those capacities, because of the lack of building up what she calls being a person, are not sufficiently integrated into herself as a source of self-esteem. This is totally different from the young woman who had capacities that she really couldn't use; one of the results of her treatment was to begin to make them available to her for her use and then for satisfaction. This person can use her capacities.

But they do not provide her with psychological sustenance. They are not a source of self-esteem for her. Why? Well she tells you the reason towards the end—because she wasn't recognized. There is this real need on the part of the mother to have an ally. Whatever the father's problems, they are really gross and flagrant. For parents who abuse their children, whether it's sexual abuse or all the other forms of abuse that are rampant, that is the most manifest part of their psychological difficulty. It is the most manifest thing that tells you that these parents are not available as a source of vitally needed recognition.

Now this brings up the difference between thinking of a self-object transference as a distortion and the self-object transference as real and welcome. The recognition that is provided becomes the source of what ultimately enables this patient to say, "What I need is recognition and that's what makes me into a person."

The imagery of the individualized self is noted by Dr. Clark throughout. Again, there is a difference in my thinking about what is defense and what is manifestation of her difficulty. Her clinging and her jumping into a new relationship right away are due to the fact that, in spite of all of her abilities, her inner feeling about herself is that she is nothing, she is not a person in and of herself.

If you address it earlier, it is even possible with a case like this that you save somebody from another disastrous marriage. Let me illustrate.

She tells you about feeling like a desert again, without a sense of direction, and she says to the therapist, "It's because I'm afraid to trust you. I'm afraid you won't point me in the right direction." The therapist says, "You begin to take care of yourself, trying to identify your feelings, and then you turn around and say you're afraid that I won't point you in the right direction." The patient complies, says it's her own laziness, etc., and she talks in the language of the therapist.

By recognizing that it is not a valid need for the therapist to take her by the hand and point her in the right direction, the therapist has the opportunity to make a genetic dynamic interpretation and reconstruction to this patient about why she clings. Why? She is now saying, "Let me cling to you," and the therapist says, "No, that's not good. You shouldn't cling to me. You should activate yourself." Instead, I'm suggesting that the therapist, who is the object of a wish to cling, now has to describe and tell the patient about that original healthy need in her childhood for recognition of what she was doing and who she was, which is what enables a child to know where she is going.

You know, the child has a sense of direction, and not just because the parent always turns her around and says go that way. The child becomes coordinated and graceful and firm and has a feeling of a sense of reality and knows where she is going because of these vital functions of being recognized as who she is when she comes home or when she goes to bed at night, instead of the kind of experience that this girl had.

This is just an example of something that both deepens

the treatment earlier and fosters the possibility of enough change early enough to avoid a disaster or a more intense transference. The patient really does cling to the therapist. That doesn't mean that the therapist does anything different, but rather that you don't keep constantly saying, "No, don't have that kind of transference to me." You say, "Yes, this is the kind of transference you have to me," and then you begin to explain it to the patient. Then, the two of you, in tandem, are going in the same direction. And you're not asking the patient to develop ego autonomy prematurely, which is, I think, what happened to this woman at the time that she made the move that led to this remarriage.

Dr. Masterson: Would it be correct to suggest, just for the sake of discussion, that you might say to her at this point something like: "It seems to me that you are feeling quite bad about yourself at the moment and impelled to turn to me to try to deal with it as a consequence of having had this experience of turning to your mother as a child and being disappointed."

Dr. Tolpin: No. It isn't that you want to tell the patient she feels bad and therefore she is impelled to turn to you, suggesting that you don't want her to turn to you, you want her to be autonomous. You do want her to turn to you. That's what you're doing there, because that is the route.

Dr. Masterson: So, what would you say? Turn it around the way you would like it.

Dr. Tolpin: I would tell the patient at this point that the experience of feeling lost was like what she had experienced when she needed recognition and that the need for recognition is important and understandable because that is what gives a sense of direction.

Dr. Masterson: But essentially, you are going to say to her that the experience of the present is basically linked, as a repetition, to experience of the past.

Dr. Tolpin: Not exactly. The past is pathological and the real reason, I think, that Dr. Masterson encourages you not to get into what he calls a regressive transference is that psychoanalysis did not sufficiently recognize, until Kohut's contribution, that what the patient repeats in many transferences are the most pathological aspects of their relationship. This idea was already in the air in the British Object Relations contributions.

This woman repeats with every man the abusive experience with a neglectful mother and an overtly abusive father. In that sense, I agree with Dr. Sifneos. And if the treatment has not mobilized this healthy aspect of the self that begins to revitalize and expand with recognition, which is really what's been behind the scenes in every therapy, then all that analysis is either useless or it is empty inside because it is the recognition that has done it.

Essentially, what I am saying to Dr. Clark, and to you, is that you should recognize it in the beginning and don't keep pushing it away. Don't make it seem as if the patient is trying to cling to you for secondary gain when what is being mobilized are those original needs for recognition that at one time in the right context were healthy needs, the need to a viable self.

Dr. Masterson: Let me address this in this way. I have no argument at all with the first part of your statement that you can do all the analytic work in the world, but if it isn't done within the framework of acknowledgment and encouragement of activation of the self, it isn't going to work. I don't have any argument with that.

But with a borderline patient, not a narcissistic one, our implicit assumption from the beginning is the acknowledgment, recognition, and support of the healthy self as the patient demonstrates it.

This does not come through transference, in my view. It comes through the therapeutic alliance as it is solidified and formed. Whether or not Dr. Clark would make an interpretation at that point would be a judgment call on her part as to how much the patient was in touch with the affect and how much of it was still being drained off by one kind of defense or another, including the clinging defense. In our experience, if you make these interpretations in a premature fashion, they lead to regression on the patient's part.

Let me put that aside for just a moment to approach this from a more general, theoretical point of view. It might have occurred to a lot of people when they first hear this case that this could be a patient who is neurotic, functions quite well, has relationships, and so forth. Therefore, the differential diagnosis between a high-level borderline personality disorder and a neurotic becomes essential. Dr. Sifneos described some excellent criteria for differentiation.

We use intrapsychic structural criteria. I think one of the advantages of this point of view that helps to make the differential diagnosis is that, if the patient is neurotic and not borderline, you will see an intrapsychic structure that explains the clinical picture. What you see is not split self and object representations, but whole self and whole object representations, both good and bad at the same time—that is, the way the patient sees herself and the way she sees the therapist.

You would also see a principal reliance on the defense mechanism of repression rather than on splitting. This would help to make the judgment that it was a neurosis and not a borderline disorder.

This case is an effort to present intensive psychoanalytic psychotherapy. What is the goal? You remember my saying the goal of confrontive psychotherapy was ego repair. You don't expect to get rid of the abandonment depression or overcome the developmental arrest. It is adaptive. You expect the patient to be able to function better, have better relationships.

The goal of this kind of treatment is not ego repair. It is the ultimate goal of working through the abandonment depression, overcoming the borderline personality disorder arrest, and putting the patient back on her developmental pathway through the oedipal stage and onward.

There are two fringe benefits to this kind of treatment which make it more than worth the effort when it can be applied. First, it eliminates the crucial vulnerability to separation stress on the part of the patient. There is separation stress in all of our lives all the time.

In addition to that, once the anchor of the abandonment depression is attenuated, the self begins to emerge quite fully. As it does, there is a kind of flowering of individuation. The patient feels as if she is becoming a new person. Actually, she is not becoming a new person. Aspects of her self that were hidden behind the depression during their development now begin to emerge and her life develops a richness and a fulfillment.

You start the treatment the same way as with confrontive therapy. The way you establish a therapeutic alliance with a borderline patient is through confrontation, whether it's confrontive therapy or analytic therapy. But as the patient establishes a therapeutic alliance, as his or her transference acting out is converted into therapeutic alliance and transference, the abandonment depression enters the scene and now the patient can work that through via memories, dreams, fantasies, and transference. At this point, the transference becomes center stage and we are able to interpret it. We don't have to confront it.

Dr. Tolpin made the point that in self psychology the aim is to foster understanding of the transference, which then leads to internalization. Well, that is more or less what we think we're doing. We are fostering internalization by working through the transference.

All this comes about within an implied assumption and recognition of acknowledgment of the self and the emergence of the self. If this patient is still in one of these marriages, which were such a prominent defense, my sense of the matter is that as the therapist tries to get to the motivation, the degree to which the patient is immersed in the defensive relationship will defeat efforts at interpretation. With borderline patients, particularly, we get very concerned about interpretation being intellectualized and producing insight as excuse, which becomes another resistance. We would like to see the insight emerge from the affect. The reason for this is very different than with a neurosis. Borderline patients remember and review memories like a motion picture projector run in reverse. They begin to remember their most recent separation stress and then they go all the way back.

For that reason, you don't ever have to interpret as much with a borderline patient as you do with a neurotic or a narcissistic patient. The patient does his own interpretations, led by the affect he is remembering and experiencing.

Let me finish by saying that I thought one of her desperate clingings to the relationships was her last line of defense against facing the hopelessness, which is a key to the abandonment depression. The hopelessness is based on facing the fact that the wish for acknowledgment from the mother for the emerging self never happened and never will happen. When that piece of abandonment depression is worked through, then you begin to get very substantial movement in the treatment.

Dr. Sifneos: I would like to very briefly, since I emphasize brief, give you an example of a patient who had that identical type of problem, but it was handled in a different way. I would be very interested to know how Dr. Masterson, as well as Dr. Tolpin, would explain that.

This was a young woman who came to us complaining of being in a battle royal with her father. She is living at home and she has an ineffectual mother. She feels that her mother never protected her from her father. Once, at the age of 13, while her mother was away, she woke up in the middle of the night and her father was in her bed fondling her genitals and her breasts.

From then on, there was a continuing battle between the two of them. Yet she stayed at home. However, when she was about 16 or 17, she went to Europe and established a relationship with a man. However, there is a difference because this was a very meaningful relationship. She wanted to get married, but felt she should ask her father's opinion. She came back to this country and, of course, her father said absolutely not.

The next year she visited another country and exactly the same thing happened. She came back and again the father discouraged her.

In follow-up, the patient emphasized two interventions as the most striking. The first one was when her therapist, a woman, said to her, "Have you realized that the reason why your father became so angry at you and you had this continuing battle was because he wanted to protect himself from doing this?" That stopped her cold because she had felt that he did it because he was really a bad person.

The second intervention that she remembered was when her therapist, with a bit of a smile, said, "I wonder why it is that you like European men and what difference the Atlantic Ocean makes. You go over there and you have meaningful relationships with men, but you cannot have relationships with American men. Is it because you want to be attached to your father who is an American man?"

The treatment lasted about five months, but the follow-

up with that woman was exceptionally fine. She had dis-
engaged herself, gone away from home, finished college,
and gotten married. There were no difficulties whatsoever.
Would you call her a neurotic facing similar types of circumstances? What is the difference?

Dr. Masterson: From my experience, yes, I'd have to call her
neurotic. I have never seen anything happen on that sort
of a short-term basis.

Dr. Sifneos: Would you say it was not splitting?

Dr. Masterson: Sometimes displacement can look like splitting
and I see displacement as a neurotic phenomenon. I cannot
conceive of it, if it were a borderline. She married an
American in this country?

Dr. Sifneos: Yes.

Dr. Masterson: Who was not older than she?

Dr. Sifneos: He was not.

Dr. Masterson: You got me. I'm mystified.

Dr. Tolpin: I had two reactions. First, we can't play duplicate
bridge in this, our therapeutic life. We never have the
same patient and so I am prepared, I'm not as hung up
about the diagnostic stuff. I am prepared to say you can
deal with focal problems and that you can deal with them
successfully with some people.

　　The second thought: I guess I found my mind wandering
which is why I can't respond effectively to the actual details. I see somebody once a week who is now in her 40s
and she came because she was thinking of divorcing her
husband. A life is very complicated. One of the things that
became apparent to me was that she really did still love
her husband. I thought that he really still loved her, but
the kind of defenses they had since a really traumatic event
in their life (for purposes of confidentiality, I won't de-

scribe it) had upset a marriage that had a pretty good equilibrium. They had been high school sweethearts and, despite their ups and downs, by modern standards I think it was a very good marriage, romantic and very satisfying sexually.

The association that led me to mention this case was that this was a very full and vital woman with a great deal of capacity to both love and to give, and with a direction in her life that was hard won. About a year into the therapy, she told me that her father had been involved with her sexually. She had never told anybody, I don't think she was especially affected by the zeitgeist because it is part of the zeitgeist now.

It made me think about the extraordinariness of what people are like and how we use this post hoc reasoning all the time. Here is a person with whom we would have used post hoc reasoning if she had had a failed marriage, a lousy sex life, and a career that went nowhere without ambitions or goals. So there are a lot more mysteries than we can explain.

Question: This is for Dr. Tolpin. In working with the borderline, where the therapist serves primarily a self-object function, especially encouraging the clinging in a therapeutic relationship . . .

Dr. Tolpin: Wait a minute. That's wrong. They don't encourage clinging in a therapeutic relationship, but they do not push the patient away who is developing a transference. It's a big difference.

Question: Perhaps take out the word *encouraging* and replace it with *acknowledging.*

Dr. Tolpin: Acknowledging, yes. It is not fostering clinging, either. There is a welcoming of a developing transference that remobilizes some normal aspects of development, as when Dr. Clark's patient said, "Point me in the right direction." That can be regarded as a remobilization—not of defensive clinging, not of pathological clinging, but of the hope for some of the things I talked about when I said the child who is recognized adequately, and grounded and anchored adequately, has a sense of direction. So, you hope the patient is going to develop more of that capacity by virtue of this transference.

Question: How would self psychology explain Dr. Masterson's predictions that under those conditions the patient would be more likely to regress when the therapist acknowledges or fosters the therapeutic relationship, the clinging—i.e., the rewarding role.

Dr. Tolpin: Dr. Masterson's idea about the rewarding unit, as I understand it, means that, in my terms, you are going along with some kind of secondary pathology. You're going along with what has happened after the self has broken down very often. I don't mean broken down in a psychotic way, but after it has not held together well and the patient does what Dr. Clark's patient does. She clings to the wreckage and uses that as her organizing focus in life. Incidentally, you probably have seen patients who collapse when they leave a bad marriage. People organize themselves around a bad marriage. As Bowlby said, it is better for an infant to have a bad home than no home at all. It is better for some people to have a bad marriage around which they are organized than no marriage at all if they lack the wherewithal to be an independent self.

You don't foster that kind of pathological relationship to the therapist, but you don't rebuff it right away.

Dr. Masterson: So how do you get around that when the patient makes such an open presentation?

Dr. Tolpin: Of what? Of a plea for a sense of direction?

Dr. Masterson: Right. You're not rebuffing them, but on the other hand you're not reinforcing them.

Dr. Tolpin: It came up in Dr. Nagel's case (Chapter I). What I said was that you don't rebuff the patient and say, "You shouldn't look to me for a sense of direction." You accept what the patient says and you recast it by explaining what you think about the request. The request means something in terms of needs that are now mobilized and of what those needs would lead the patient to feel like. The patient would feel grounded, for example, if you say, "I understand why you want me to give you a sense of direction." You're not giving the patient a sense of direction when you say that. Rather, you are explaining that the therapist, as the idealized self-object now, makes the patient feel strong, with a sense of direction if that relationship is working. You explain something about that in terms of the patient's development as a child and how that was disrupted.

I think there is a disagreement now between us. You keep making it sound as if I'm saying, "Yes, honey, come sit on my lap and I'll give you a sense of direction."

Dr. Masterson: I think you are. When the patient says "Tell me something, do something for me," you are going to act in response to this initiative. But then you're going to say this is not a response to and a reinforcement of that initiative because your act takes place only in form of words. I think that's a contradiction in terms.

Let me make this clear. I don't have any basic argument about this with a narcissistic disorder. We would make an interpretation along those lines, without much reservation. But not with a borderline patient. This is, I think, the key to our difference and that is what we think heals.

Obviously, we also accept the clinging, but we analyze it, we investigate it, because our basic assumption is that what's requiring them to cling and not allowing their self-capacities to develop is the abandonment depression that lies underneath. If we can get them to work that through, what you think will happen through self-object functions will happen through working through the depression. When you intervene with a borderline patient in response to the clinging, you are reversing the direction.

Dr. Tolpin: I think this is getting into quibbling. Your therapies last as long as our therapies because it takes an enormous amount of time to change self-organization and to really acquire some of the capacities that people need.

I think this ought to be a point at which we understand that the frameworks are different, that what I think you mean by abandonment depression is the structural deficit, and that the time that is taken to work through abandonment depression in your framework is the time it takes for enough transmuting internalization to take place so patients actually feel they have enough capacities of their own to change from this self-state of a desert that's dry and empty to the self-state of a person with some life who finds something beautiful—herself.

Question: I need a point of clarification from Dr. Tolpin. If I understand you correctly, you're saying that you acknowledge the need that is happening in the transference acting out.

Dr. Tolpin: It isn't acting out in the transference. It is remobilizing that need to a point where it is being accepted and can be in the room between the two of us.

Question: What you're acknowledging, then, is the healthy, original need. You don't want to discourage the patient because you would be devitalizing the original impulse towards health.

Dr. Tolpin: That's right, you don't want to discourage it because it's that need and its understanding and wording in the transference which is inevitable. You do not have to try to thwart it because it will be thwarted, I assure you. It is that need and its growth in a self-object unit that makes the actual change possible. You don't want to rebuff it or stunt it again, because that is really what happened in the development of these kids. The parents needed them to be precocious, for example. The parents needed them as the self-object for themselves, as this mother did. Some parents will do anything to keep the peace. They are so exhausted and depleted themselves. The father goes for the kid. Wonderful. The mother doesn't have to deal with him.

Question: So you're saying that interpreting the need doesn't necessarily encourage more acting out. Forgive me for using the words *acting out*, which are more behavioral. What's the word you use, behavior?

Dr. Tolpin: It is *remobilized*. It is the experience of, "Oh, I have this valid need and it can be directed toward this person who is an echo of what I need."

Question: So you're saying it doesn't encourage regression.

Dr. Tolpin: That's right. Properly understood, it doesn't encourage regression because, contrary to what Dr. Masterson said, it is not an encouragement to regressively sit on your lap. It is the possibility that the person will feel more alive and less desiccated. She doesn't feel like a desert as much, because she now has this internal experience of a need that is valid, that is responded to with recognition.

Question: This is a question I'd like to address to all discussants today. Do you accept the force of the unconscious and its effect on behavior in formulating your theoretical framework? If so, what is its role in your treatment?

Dr. Tolpin: It's a very good question because it is clear, as Dr. Sifneos' work dramatically illustrates, that there is a difference in thinking about what is unconscious, what is defended against. I don't think any psychoanalyst or psychoanalytically oriented therapist has changed the view about the power of the unconscious. However, the view about what is unconscious and what the defenses are against is vastly changed.

The whole gamut of therapies that focus on relationships have fundamentally changed the view of what is central in a problem from the oedipal problem to something else. For example, in Dr. Clark's case, it is the need for recognition. That does change your views about the unconscious.

Dr. Masterson: I agree that everybody accepts the force of the unconscious. As far as personality disorders are concerned, what is far more important is that these complexes are not unconscious, but that they are kept separated. They are conscious, but they are kept separated from each other by splitting. When the splitting is overcome, they emerge.

This is one of the reasons, by the way, that interpretation with borderlines is not the effective agent. Interpretation was developed to deal specifically with the fact that the conflict was unconscious. It was a conflict between an unconscious, let's say, id force and a super ego force, not available to the ego. Therefore, the ego couldn't deal with it. The way to solve the problem was to make an interpretation to the ego of what the unconscious force was and then the ego would rearrange the forces. That is not the way treatment works with borderline and narcissistic disorders. Therefore, that aspect of it does not play such an important part.

Dr. Sifneos: It is preconscious for the neurotics, not deeply unconscious, but somewhat preconscious,

Question: Dr. Tolpin, I want to go back to the patient's need for recognition. Would you ever, under any circumstances, see that as defensive? Or do you always see it as coming from a healthy aspect of the real self?

Dr. Tolpin: The patient Dr. Klein presented this morning clamors noisily for recognition of his grandiose self, as Dr. Klein called it and what in my way of thinking is pathological grandiosity. So, indeed, the demand for recognition of that would be a way of maintaining the self that the patient has constituted and that is part of what the work is. The defenses don't mean that you're warding off something, as in original theory or a nuclear oedipal problem. They mean you're trying to preserve what you've got and you can't let go of it without assistance.

Yes, that's a perfect example of the clamor for recognition. "Look at me, look how terrific I am." It is something that you have to understand in the workings of the mind in order to understand that that is not the "real self." That is a pathological formation. At the same time, you have to understand that that is how this person held himself together. It wasn't brought out, interestingly enough, that there really was a very significant precipitant. I think self psychology probably emphasizes much more the dynamics of the present illness and the precipitants in the present illness. Very often, they are a really significant clue as to what some of the dynamics and genetics of the personality are.

This man, amongst other things, lost an admiring, admired boss, which is a precipitation of his father's disillusion and his panic about his own possible disillusion. While you would recognize that this man's defensive grandiosity holds him together, you still do not respond to that as though it is a valid claim of a little boy for recognition from his father.

PART II

Workshops

9

Workshop

James F. Masterson, M.D.

Dr. Masterson: I'd like to run this workshop like an enlarged continuous case seminar. Yesterday was our turn to describe what we do. Today is your turn. The floor is open to questions, case vignettes, or fuller case presentations. I will free associate to what the therapist presents so as to provide contrasts and comparisons with the field in general. I don't believe that people learn by identification with the aggressor. My function is not to put you down, but to try to help you understand what's going on so you can do better.

Question: Would you elaborate on your view of self psychology?

Dr. Masterson: First, their conception of psychopathology revolves strictly around defects in the structure of the self. They do not subscribe to the idea of diagnosis other than of the structures of the self. As far as they are concerned, there is no such thing as a borderline personality disorder that differs from a narcissistic personality disorder. They are both disorders of the self with the structural defects in the self.

The problem with that point of view was illustrated yesterday, by the differences in the therapeutic approach of Dr. Nagel and Dr. Klein. With the diagnostic approach, you use confrontation with a borderline and you use interpretation with a narcissistic disorder. It is diagnosis that tells you which one to use.

Therefore, if the self psychology therapists are going to view borderline patients as the same as narcissistic patients and use the same interpretative approach, it won't work.

It doesn't work because the interpretation steps into the rewarding unit projection and resonates with the patient's wish to be taken care of. Therapeutic movement stops.

One of the difficulties that plagues this field, which we don't see in the physical sciences, is the fact that in the one-to-one interaction with patients there are many many things you can do from which will come change. So the fact that somebody changes by himself is no proof of anything, other than that he changes for some strange reason.

The self psychology therapist will get a kind of behavioral change based on the patient's compliance with the therapist's taking the rewarding unit role.

I have some experimental evidence. It comes out most clearly in the people we supervise, who always seem to start off using interpretation with borderline patients, but the patient doesn't start to move until we get them switched to confrontation.

In essence, the self psychology view seems to be that all of these disorders, including neurosis, are basically problems in the structure of the self. Therefore, all the rest of psychoanalytic theory is inappropriate. I think self psychologists don't see the problem as trying to accommodate one view with another view, but rather as one where they have the correct view and we don't understand it. As a result, it is not a matter of education, but a matter of resistance.

I think that is their basic assumption and it is breathtaking, to say the least. There is less dispute about the treatment of the narcissistic disorder since both our treatments have similar, although not the same results.

Question: Do the self psychologists use DSM-III?

Dr. Masterson: They don't use DSM-III, at all. They don't use object relations theory, at all. That is why they give such grudging acknowledgment to these points of view. They talk about the structure of the self. It took me years, reading Kohut and the other self psychologists to understand the language. Dr. Tolpin says: "Kohut's greatest discovery was the recognition that the mother's inability to function as a self object for the child resulted in the child having trouble in functioning as a self for himself." This is the same point of view as the one I described: "The mother's inability to acknowledge the child's individuation produces a developmental arrest and then all the other difficulties follow."

I don't think that was his greatest discovery. I think his greatest discovery was the term "self-object." The reason I think that is that I have been through some of the same route. I recognized that the mother's inability to acknowledge the self resulted in difficulties of the self. What better theory could there be than object relations theory to deal with that? When Kohut made the same observation, he was at a crossroads: either to follow object relations theory, which would have placed him in the mainstream with his peers or to invent the term "self-object," which seems to me a very artificial term. Why couldn't you have the acknowledgment of the self intrapsychically as one of the functions of the object? This gives rise to the developmental experience.

At one of these conferences in Los Angeles in 1980, a therapist mentioned to me that she was treating a borderline patient and had a self psychology supervisor. She was very unhappy with the patient's lack of improvement and asked if I would be willing to supervise her and a group of other therapists in the same situation?

What I did basically was to convert them from what Dr. Klein was doing to what Dr. Nagel was doing. The patients picked up immediately and started to change.

This demonstrates the key clinical difference. There is, however, a deeper difference which plagues me, as it must plague you.

What did Kohut mean by structures of the self? I finally figured out that it means the capacities. Not structures, but capacities for self-assertion, for self-soothing, to maintain self-esteem. All of these are capacities of the self and, therefore, what they evaluate is the degree to which these capacities are impaired.

The other thing they evaluate is the way the patient relates to them, which brings up the other issue that perplexes the field. This is the way they get around the fact that it's not transference, but transference acting out, by using this wonderful term "self-object transference."

In certain ways it is a very attractive theory. It is coherent, it is inclusive. I can see the degree of appeal it has for people in this field, especially if they have no other grounding.

I entered the field by studying first the borderline personality disorder and then I came to the narcissistic disorder and had some trouble learning and understanding it, particularly the closet narcissistic disorder, because they're not exhibitionistic and can't maintain the continuous activation of the defense. Unless, as with Klein's case, you use the proper interventions, you never find out that what looks to you like clinging is really the search for you to mirror their grandiosity. In other words, the grandiosity doesn't come out unless you have the right approach. And so they look like borderlines. I think that we confronted them for some time and thought these were untreatable borderlines. Have you noticed how many papers begin,

"These difficult-to-treat patients. . . ." I often wonder how many of the authors are treating closet narcissists as borderline? No wonder they're difficult. I think that was an error we made until we finally got around to understanding the closet narcissistic personality disorder.

I am trying now to explain how it is that self psychologists maintain that the borderline is the same as the narcissistic disorder when everybody else sees the borderline as different. Since the closet narcissistic disorder so mimics the borderline, they have made the reverse mistake that we made. They look at the borderline and they think it is a closet narcissistic disorder.

I think Dr. Tolpin did say that the big thing about what Kohut did and I did was to get away from classical instinctual theory and oedipal conflict, and get back to the pre-oedipal, as well as to real-life events that occurred in development as opposed to the child's fantasies.

Question: The self psychology view reminds me of Kleinian thinking where the mother and anything else outside the child don't matter. The child has this kind of genetic firmness that unfolds and flowers within unless the environment is too bad. That is the kind of imagery I'm getting— that treatment is "be nice." At a clinical presentation by a self psychologist, I asked him what was the distinction between his empathic perspective, which he called unique to this treatment, and the usual clinical approach.

Dr. Masterson: In his case presentation, did he describe exactly what he said to the patient?

Question: Yes. It was something like "Oh, you must have felt very bad."

Dr. Masterson: Mirroring without the interpretation.

Question: No interpretation other than he's holding court. He was very honest about it. I then asked him, "Can you draw a distinction between what you're doing and the usual containment of the projective identification and gradually working it out?" He said, "No, it's exactly the same."

Dr. Masterson: I share your perspective about Melanie Klein's view that the mother is a kind of unnecessary baggage whose function may be to modify and moderate the child's aggression, at most. But everything else is genetic and everything else is aggression. Many of Klein's clinical observations were extremely innovative and we still use them today—the splitting defense, the depressive position, etc. But the views of the self psychologists are really not the same. They are trying to get away from object relations theory, so they stay away from intrapsychic structure and end up with descriptive terms. They call it the self-object function of the parent. That is what I call the parent's capacity to acknowledge and support the child's individuation, or emerging self.

Thus, unlike the Kleinians who see that as a very peripheral tangential function that just helps the child moderate his aggression, the self psychologists see it, as I do, as vital for the development of the self.

Dr. Tolpin says the self-object functions of the parent are vital for the child. Every child's self, as it emerges, goes through crises. That makes for the usual physical analogy—the child falls down, skins his knee, cries, is unhappy, and the mother says, "There, there, that's going to be all right." The psychological analogy is that it is inevitable in normal development for the child to go through these crises.

From my developmental point of view, an analogy would be in the rapprochement stage, when it is inevitable that the child's grandiosity and omnipotence will go through phase-appropriate frustration.

In their view, the self-object function of the parent when the child is having one of these crises of self is to understand and respond, to lend a psychological hand. This heals that crisis. And then, every time a crisis is healed, the self is strengthened and the capacity to manage, to assert, to soothe, begins to grow and consolidate and become cohesive. That is their basic developmental frame.

You have to understand, by the way, that Kohut had a developmental theory without any study of development, without any reference to development except as it was reported on the analytic couch. So you can imagine the reaction of the self psychologists when Daniel Stern's book was published (*The First Relationship: Mother and Infant.* Harvard U. Press, 1977). He had filled in this hole that had been ignored.

To follow the implications of that view of development for treatment, Dr. Tolpin says that the therapist in the transference provides a new self-object function and that the way the therapist performs that function is to listen, to understand and explain. The patient's fragmented self feels a fit, which it did not feel as a child, and it is this fit that enables the patient to consolidate himself.

It sounds to me as if they are saying that transference cures, that countertransference cures. You can see how useful this term self-object is because, by using it to qualify the term transference, they never face the issue that I stress about the difference between transference acting-out and therapeutic alliance and the importance of this difference for treatment.

The key issue can be clearly illustrated through the idealizing transference. They accept the idealization. There is a long way between accepting idealization and promoting idealization, and I have a strong suspicion that they promote it. This raises the other paramount issue, from my perspective—their conception of therapeutic neutrality. I don't understand this because, if the idea is that the transference cures and all you have to do is listen and get it right, get whatever the patient's pain at the moment is and explain it to him since what matters is the emotional experience of the patient, reality or not, then therapeutic neutrality is irrelevant.

Question: What is your view of therapeutic neutrality?

Dr. Masterson: It's a life preserver to protect the patient and the therapist from being overwhelmed by the patient's projections and the therapist's countertransference. The therapist does not have a personal relationship with the patient, nor does he permit personal things about him to be told to the patient. The therapist does not do things in reality for the patient except therapeutic interventions. As an offshoot of that, the therapist has to be 100% for adaptation. But it seems to me that is realistic, if not neutral. So that our stance is 100% reality in terms of adaptation and neutrality. For example, a borderline patient may want you to take over for him. You do not do it. You remain neutral so you can analyze this wish.

Question: Does neutrality mean sitting there, saying nothing?

Dr. Masterson: No, no.

Question: Talking?

Dr. Masterson: Yes. I can tell you a little story that defines it. This friend of mine did a study of psychotherapy. He got a computer, he hooked it up with a galvanometer, and connected the wires to the palms of the patient's hands. When the patient talked, the palm reflex, through perspiration, would turn the computer on. The patient would say something and begin to perspire. The computer would be silent for a while and then it would say, "What you were talking about seemed very interesting. Maybe you should go back to it."

My friend commented, "Not only can this apparatus do psychotherapy, it can also do psychoanalysis with only two modifications: You pull a blank screen down in front of it and pull out the plug." This kind of blankness is not what I mean. You could tell from the way I talk about the clinical material and from those presentations. We are 100% behind health and adaptation.

Question: Aren't we supposed to be interested in the patient?

Dr. Masterson: In one of my books, I emphasize that I don't mean that one should be a block of wood. You have to be interested in your patient. You must be emotionally involved in the treatment. I also make the point that you must acknowledge for the patient his reality triumphs and sympathize with his failures. You have to be a human being. I am thinking about not stepping into the patient's projections when I use the word neutrality.

Question: Are you then like a totally non-critical parent?

Dr. Masterson: No, you're not a parent.

Question: Under no circumstances am I going to criticize you or judge you?

Dr. Masterson: Yes, your position is not to judge. You often have to mention this.

Question: Is it therapeutic neutrality which enables my patient to work with me?

Dr. Masterson: To me, that's only the beginning because it doesn't cover what you do about all of the patient's efforts to get you to do things for him.

Question: That is a judgment. So, we're really not talking about not making judgments? You make a correct judgment—a matter of stepping in with a stand for mental health, planning a background with a healthy result and object.

Dr. Masterson: It's called therapeutic neutrality. It's not neutral neutrality, it's therapeutic neutrality. If you've got a better word, I'd be happy to use it. But the biggest problem people have in doing this work is exactly that. What I mean is taking what I call a therapeutically neutral stance towards all the patient's projections. He says, "You look bored today. You look like you're tired." "Well, what makes you ask that?" "Why is it you don't smile when I come in? You never tell me what to do." All of these are projections of the rewarding unit on the therapist; some of them are far more subtle than that.

Most of the work I do in supervision is helping therapists understand how you use therapeutic neutrality to deal with these projections. You *reflect* them rather than *react* to them.

Question: Can you comment on the statistical data, if any, on results presented by self psychologists?

Dr. Masterson: Dr. Sifneos described yesterday his follow-up studies. I did a follow-up study. I first did the psychotherapy research study of treatment of the borderline adolescent. Then, I followed them up seven years later.

The self-psychologists would say now, I think, that it's too early and that they are just getting around to that. But my guess is that it works, even with a narcissistic disorder. Does it work to make him object-related? I don't think so. When it works, I think the structure of self comes together and the patient begins to recognize that there are other people out there and that if he wants his narcissistic goals, he'd better find some way of getting along with them. This is not the same as being object-related.

Question: I understand the difference between the borderline and the narcissist. But how do you deal with an extremely acting-out narcissist without getting the backlash that you get when you confront?

Dr. Masterson: That is a very good question. First, however, let me make an addendum to the question I was answering. This idea of saying to the patient, "Oh, I know this feels terrible. It's an awful thing," is a kind of mirroring that is exactly what they're looking for if it's a narcissistic disorder. It would be like saying to a borderline patient, "Let me take over for you and let me tell you what to do." I hope you noticed, in Dr. Klein's presentation that there was no mirroring without interpretation. One of the reasons our approach is similar to the self-psychology approach is the nature of the disorder. There is only one way you're going to get access to the narcissistic patient: you've got to go through the narcissistic window. That's the only way.

That is why we call it mirroring interpretation of narcissistic vulnerability. If you say to a patient, "You seem exquisitely vulnerable to other people's responses," the patient will love it: "Somebody finally understands me." But you step into that omnipotent object that makes him feel special and wonderful and grandiose; as a result, there's no movement.

There's nothing in clinical work that's black and white. Patients run into terrible situations and you certainly have to say something—"It must have been very difficult," and so forth. And there are certain stages of treatment where the patient is in very bad shape.

The interpretation will get the patient to begin to explore his narcissistic vulnerability. When you've got him exploring, you have established a therapeutic alliance. The patient's explorations will lead him to discover that what he thought was wrong with all you folks is actually his grandiose expectations.

To answer the other question: The narcissistic disorder patient, who has a lot of acting-out defenses, has a poor prognosis because, in order to deal with him, you have to confront the acting out. There is no other therapeutic technique I know of to deal with acting out but confrontation. However, you have to realize that you are exposing his narcissistic vulnerability when you're confronting the acting out, so you have to do a two-step process. You confront the acting out and then you make the mirroring narcissistic interpretation. That is why it is so difficult, and that is why the prognosis is not as good.

Question: You referred yesterday to the higher-level borderline, not talking about somebody on the border of psychosis. I'm wondering why that term "borderline" is used.

Dr. Masterson: It's how it originated. Like so many things, it's historical. The whole notion of the borderline personality disorder arose not in psychiatric circles, but in psychoanalytic circles. They had these people on the couch who were functioning pretty well and they were trying to analyze them. The first thing they knew, the patients had a psychotic attack, which would then restore. Thus, they thought at the time that these patients were closer to psychosis than they were to neurosis, even though they looked like they were neurotic. That is why they put them on the borderline in between.

The problems of introducing a new term are far greater than the problems of redefining an old term. We left the old term, but we paid a big price because we have since learned that the spectrum of the borderline personality is extremely wide and there are an enormous number of high-level borderlines who function extremely well in their occupation. They have trouble with object relations. However, they look very neurotic and are being treated as neurotics by many analysts.

The other price is even bigger. The lay literature on the borderline is a disaster, always talking about the lower-level borderline: They can't function, they use drugs, they use alcohol, they're very difficult or impossible to treat. As a result, when people read this and then find out they have a borderline diagnosis, they fall into despair.

I was in Denver doing a conference. Two psychoanalysts from the Denver Psychoanalytic Institute came to the conference and were utterly shocked. They said that if they make a borderline diagnosis, they send the patient to somebody else as these patients are not treatable.

Question: Whatever happened to pseudoneurotic schizophrenia?

Dr. Masterson: That's it! Such terms as pseudoneurotic schizophrenia or ambulatory schizophrenia were applied to lower-level borderlines who had separation psychosis. Upper-level borderlines never have psychosis, for good reason, since their ego is too strong.

We talk about difficulty. It is not always that difficult to diagnose once you understand that there are some patients at the upper level that are hard to differentiate between borderline and neurotic and there are some at the lower level that are harder to differentiate between psychotic and borderline; those in between are not that difficult.

I would like to say, here, that I had a fantastic reaction to Dr. Sifneos' lecture because he did just what I had hoped for: to show the difference between the personality disorder and the neurotic. He described it perfectly. We can describe the difference as follows: A patient comes in, a neurotic patient, and he is talking about something and you make an observation about what he is talking about. You schedule another session and he comes back and says, "You know, I was thinking about what you said and I got a little anxious and I went to bed and I had this dream and these are my thoughts about the dream."

A borderline patient comes in and you make an observation. About 100 things could happen and none of them will be what I described for the neurotic. He may not hear you, he may object to what you said, he may fight, he may stalk out of the office, he may not come back. If he comes back, he may not remember.

What are we talking about? We're talking about the fact that at the outset of treatment you have a therapeutic alliance with a neurotic, but you don't with a borderline. The first therapeutic goal with a borderline is to achieve a therapeutic alliance.

Now, theoretically, why do you have a therapeutic alliance? The dialogue between Dr. Sifneos and myself yesterday was all about this and about the effect on therapeutic interventions, as well as on observations. When I do the developmental lecture, I use a diagram of how the self and object representations develop. Before you get to the rapprochement stage, you have split self and object representations in normal development. Following that stage, the split self and object representations come together as wholes—whole self, good and bad, whole object, good and bad.

The clinical significance of that is that splitting disappears, its place is taken by repression, and the capacity for what we call whole object relations emerges—the capacity to relate to you as you are in reality, a therapist, as well as to see his projections upon you, to see your bad parts as well as your good parts at the same time.

In *Psychotherapy of the Borderline Adult*, I described a case I treated not too long after I got out of training. I saw the patient three times a week. I thought he was an anxiety hysteric, I did some fancy interpretations, and he seemed to get a little better. After 18 months he stopped. About 15 years later when I got into this work, I was very regretful because I realized he was a hysterical borderline and I really hadn't done what I should have. And then, lo and behold, he walks back into my office. He had been divorced twice, was paying alimony to two women and going with a third woman who was demanding marriage. He said he certainly couldn't afford to pay alimony to three women, so he would try treatment instead. I said I thought that was a good idea.

I now treated him as a hysterical borderline and the difference in the result was the difference between night and day. The way you tell the difference is as follows: You must take the patient where he is when he comes in. You confront his defenses. If he integrates the confrontations, he is going to go into an abandonment depression and mother will emerge on center stage. If he is a hysterical neurotic, there won't be an abandonment depression when you get through the defenses. The patient will probably become more anxious and sex and mother and father will emerge on center stage.

Let me describe an upper-level borderline patient where the therapist has gone along a little too much with patient's acting out through an affair. This relationship is not what it appears to be. It is a defense, not a genuine effort at a real relationship. Although the man is a better candidate than any she's had before in her life, he's still a defense against treatment. The patient, in her development, went from mother to father to deal with her abandonment depression. She is now going from the therapist to this man to deal with the abandonment depression about the mother that's emerging. And she's not going to come to grips with that until the therapist confronts the acting out.

PARTICIPANT'S CASE REPORT NO. 1

Participant: The patient is in her late 40s and I've been seeing her for three years. She's on public assistance, has training as a surgical nurse, but has not worked in many years. I met her in a hospital. Before that, most of her 20 years as a psychiatric patient were spent in and out of hospitals. She would call the emergency room, saying, "I'm going to kill myself." Early on, she did make several suicide attempts. She actually has not made one for quite a long time.

Dr. Masterson: She really meant to kill herself?

Participant: I don't think so.

Dr. Masterson: It's very important to differentiate between a manipulative attempt and a serious effort at suicide. If people want to kill themselves, generally there are serious signs. They had an adequate dose of whatever they took, they fell unconscious, they are in the ICU for a number of days. These are the people who meant to kill themselves. It's extremely important to differentiate between the two because if the suicide attempt is a manipulative weapon, you're going to have to handle that right away.

Participant: Actually, most of her attempts seemed to me to be much more like self-mutilation, although some of it had some pretty serious consequences. Once she drank some caustic solution and gave herself problems with her throat. It had been 10 years since her last attempt when I saw her.

She had had every diagnosis known to man. It often seems as if that's one of the hallmark things you learn on the phone: "I've been diagnosed schizophrenic and everything in DSM." She had had every pill, plus 200 or more shock treatments.

The background of this particular session was that she was having a problem with her medical assistance in paying for the treatment. They had decided they were not going to pay for it except for every other week or month. This was after two years in which I had been able to arrange with them to cover treatment every week plus 12 or 15 other sessions during that period.

She was very upset by this and I had said that I would help her with the appeal process, but that in the meantime she was going to have to be responsible for a certain amount. So we set a very low fee that she had to pay. I wasn't going to do the treatment for free.

She had been quite angry with me in the preceding session because I would not commit myself as to what I would do if they stopped the coverage. I said I would not decide one way or another until we got all the facts. We would have to talk more about this.

She's angry. This is a person who also has lots of trouble with her medical caregivers. She goes to see them all the time, calls them all the time, insists on pills. They give pills to her until they can't stand her anymore and then they throw her out of the office.

So she came in talking about how all these doctors wouldn't treat her because she's a mental patient and doctors don't want to see mental patients. "It's a conspiracy to get rid of us," she said.

We had previously noted that when she was in that kind of haranguing mode about her medical caregiver, she usually was talking about me. So I said, "It seems like you're avoiding something you're mad about at me." She denied it and said, "You always say that we have to talk about my part in what happens with these doctors and I don't want to do that because I don't have any part in it."

She continued, "I'm just a victim. I've always been a victim everywhere I go, basically." I said, "As we've previously noted, there's not anything we can do about your doctors in this office, or about society, and I'm wondering why you're not wanting to talk about what you are doing or not doing."

At that point she got up out of her chair. This patient had always had a tendency to walk around in my office as a defense whenever things got really hot. We had spent about a year on that. So she got up and started walking around, pacing, looking out the window. I said, "Again it seems like you're avoiding the issue of talking to me in words and you're trying to communicate with me in actions, but it isn't working."

She sat down after I told her to and then began to focus on me. "What is the matter with you? I am a sick person. I come here because there is something wrong with me and you are supposed to fix me." She pushes me into a kind of silence, sometimes, with these rageful outbursts. This was one of those times where I was taken aback by all this rage and her repeating, "You have to help me. Tell me what to do. I don't know what to do."

I was silent for a while and wondering how I would get into this. I know this is happening, as it always does, and ask myself why I am always sitting there with this. Finally, I said to her, "It seems to me that you're conceiving of this treatment as a kind of Heloise's Hints or something where I'm supposed to tell you what to do and then you're going to do it and everything is going to be all great and fine."

Well, she stared at me as if I were from Mars. She was quiet for a second and then she just burst into this uncontrollable laughter. She started just laughing and laughing and laughing. And I'm sitting there and I'm thinking, I'm still kind of shell-shocked. This patient really evokes that in me more than almost anybody else because I'm thinking that in about five seconds she's going to switch over and start screaming at me again.

It was toward the end of the hour by that time. She actually stopped and said, "You know, I wish I had your confidence." And I didn't know what to say to that and I often have all kinds of problems knowing how to respond to this patient's, "You got to fix me." It makes a sort of sense to me when I get caught up in it. I'm here to fix her and she's there for me to fix her, not for her to work on herself. So it seems like she brought up a lot of the issues we were talking about concerning taking responsibility. So that's why I presented her.

Dr. Masterson: Well, what are you feeling with her while all this is going on? You'd like to shoot her?

Participant: That's probably the predominant feeling like, "Oh, why did I take on this person?"

Dr. Masterson: I think what we try to do here, if we can get control of our own anger, is to take a step back and try to figure out, theoretically first, what is going on here. What is this patient doing, how would you, could you, figure out theoretically what she is doing?

Participant: I thought that she was probably trying to put me, alternately into the rewarding unit, then the withdrawing unit.

Dr. Masterson: Absolutely. She's got it right. What life is about is that you're supposed to be the rewarding unit; and if you're not the rewarding unit, she's entitled to treat you as the withdrawing unit. Correct? Now, does somebody else want to say what he or she would do with this patient under these conditions?

Question: Perhaps she has already set boundaries? I don't see any limit-setting structure at all in terms of we have to do this and to do that and you can't do this and you can't do that and if you do, this session is over.

Participant: Actually, I do have a lot of strict arrangements about many things, but less so about the moment-to-moment things. A lot of it has to do with what I will and won't do with regard to hospital treatment of her and phone calls and all that kind of business. Not so much within the hour.

Dr. Masterson: Once in a while, with a patient who is acting out like this, I will tell about this cartoon. This skinny little patient is huddling in the chair and looming over him is this giant figure of a psychiatrist. The caption says, "Mr. Smith, the reason you feel inferior is you are inferior."

Another idea I have had is that the borderline patient transference acts out with such intensity and such an air of reality that the therapist sometimes feels caught up between humane consideration for the patient and doing therapy. This therapist is already caught up in counter-transference. So, this patient's way of dealing with her problems is, "I'm going to push the environment around as I see fit, as long as I want, in order not to have to deal with my problems." You're in trouble because she's also on public assistance. Why can't this woman work?

Participant: We argue about that because I don't believe there is any reason.

Dr. Masterson: Did you tell her that?

Participant: Yes.

Dr. Masterson: It's a beautiful example of how flagrant the acting-out gets. What is often missed is that you must escalate your confrontation to the degree of acting-out. If you don't, you don't make it. I get consultations where therapists claim confrontation is not working. I see the patient and what has happened is that the acting-out is far worse than the therapist realized and he hasn't been escalating the confrontation.

I have another little story I use to illustrate this with a patient whom I've been confronting and confronting, but who is not integrating it. I say, have you heard the story of this man walking down the country road who sees this farmer who is hitting a mule over the head with a wooden 2 × 4. The guy runs up to the farmer and says, "Stop that! You're going to hurt this mule!" The farmer says, "No, no, I'm just trying to get his attention." Then I'll say to the patient, "I've used all my 2 × 4s on you and I'm still not getting your attention." That sounds like a terrible thing to say, and it is, unless it's appropriate to the situation.

You're behind the 8-ball when the patient is on public assistance to begin with. She's already got the environment to gratify her. You reinforce rewarding unit projections and they take on a greater and greater air of reality. When you saw her for a lower fee, she said to you, "What are you going to do?" If that happened to me, I would be so shocked I'd fall off my chair. What do you mean by what am I going to do? What does it have to do with me? Why are you asking me what I'm going to do? I'm not going to do anything. What are *you* going to do?

You've got to counter her point by point. With this patient, you can use words. Of course, they have to be appropriate to the clinical situation. You could say, "If stubbornness were a virtue, you'd be sitting at the right hand of God. You are so determined to force me and everybody else in the world to take care of you, or otherwise you're entitled to be mad at the whole universe as a way of dealing with your problems. I don't know why you come and see me. You don't want to deal with your problems. What are you doing here?"

You have been intimidated by this patient in two ways. You're intimidated by the pseudoreality of a rewarding unit projection and you're frightened of her rage. I'm not frightened of her rage.

Participant: I don't think I am, really. I mean, what's the worst that can happen? She could walk out.

Dr. Masterson: Maybe that's it. That's the worst that could happen, she could walk out. That could be the *best* that could happen.

Participant: She'll never do that, I think.

Dr. Masterson: "She'll never do that." You've got her until the grave, is that it? Unless you start doing the work here, that may be the situation.

Question: That should be done when the patient is first seen.

Dr. Masterson: Of course, from the outset, from the first phone call, from the first session.

Question: Once you realize that . . . and it's been going on for a while, how can you get yourself out?

Dr. Masterson: You have to realize that in a clinical setting, these patients have the whole clinic reinforcing their projections. The whole system reinforces them. So, how do you get out of it? That depends on how deeply you've gotten in; sometimes you can't get out if you've gotten in too deeply. In other words, if you resonated with a resistance too deeply and too long, sometimes you just can't get out.

But the way you get out is to say to the patient, however you yourself want to do it, "I've been reviewing the notes (or I've been to a conference) and the way we have been working is not productive or in your best interest, so I'm going to change." You have to let them know you're changing for *your* reasons and not their reasons.

Then, you could continue, "I know you're unhappy with me and what's going on here. Now let me tell you, I am unhappy with you and what's going on here. It seems to me that what you are doing not only with me but in your life is you are insisting that somebody else do for you what nobody can do for you but yourself. Then, when it doesn't happen and you try to manipulate people into doing it, including me, you feel entitled to this rage when it doesn't come about.

"I think the reason you're doing it is to try to avoid the rage that's inside. You're going to have to stop doing it and come to grips with that rage with me in this session if we are to continue. That is what the treatment is about."

If the patient wants to scream and be as angry as they want to be in the office, that doesn't bother me very much, even if they're mad at me. If it's directed and it's out in the open, it's something you can get a hold of.

You're going to have to tell this to this patient of yours.

And you're going to have to be very firm. What's going to happen is that she may say, "Thank God somebody finally figured out what I'm doing." But then she's going to start to test. You'll get phone calls: "I've got to see you." "I can't see you. I'll see you at the next session." You hold your position. Her test is going to be: Do I really have to manage these feelings myself? And your answer constantly has to be yes, otherwise we have no work together.

PARTICIPANT'S CASE REPORT NO. 2

Participant: Our group focuses on co-dependence, using a child within model, which is how I came to hear what somebody called the buzz word of co-dependence. I thought this concept needs some underpinning. Your view explores dependence as well as Adult Children of Alcoholics (ACOA) issues.

The patient's attendance at individual sessions has been regular, but her group attendance is more sporadic, because her getting to group involves her in conflict within her family. Also, her attitude towards other group members is full of projections that depend on current life events.

Mrs. B. came to our agency at the suggestion of a friend she met at AA meetings. She said her reason for coming was "to find out who I am and why I act the way I do and why I think the way I do." She had been in counseling several times, but had never been able to stick to it. She was 43 when she came. She decided to leave the last counselor because she had told her to leave her husband and she said she couldn't stand that. She'd been hospitalized with a nervous breakdown once around 1980 as a consequence of her drinking. She said that they had diagnosed her as borderline, and she didn't like that word. I said, "That's okay. Don't worry about it, we won't use it here."

Her husband was at that time in an alcohol rehab unit and he had recently clashed with one of the rehab counselors during a family weekend where she had felt blamed and exluded by him. Mrs. B. is a housewife who hasn't worked regularly since she met her husband. I think she worked on Wall Street.

Dr. Masterson: How long had he been in the unit before she came for treatment?

Participant: He was in the middle of a 28-day rehab.

Dr. Masterson: He had been there 14 days? Did that have something to do with her coming? Was it the precipitating stress?

Participant: Yes, that would be it, the abandonment, the separation.

Dr. Masterson: Not only his physical leaving, but because they're probably confronting him and he's getting mad and he's coming home and dumping it on her, or dumping it on her when she visits.

Participant: Yes! The visit was not great. She was blamed. She has two older sons, 20 and 19, who live at home and go to work with her husband, who is a construction worker. She also has a teenage daughter and a younger son. She characterizes her older sons as too dependent on her, unwilling to move out and fend for themselves. She says they're verbally abusive, which they are. Everybody screams at everybody. When you call there, you can really hear it. And her husband refuses to discipline them.

They have been married since 1967. Mrs. B. is an active alcoholic and had abused alcohol for two years until 1983 when she stopped and began to attend AA. She had had two slips, both connected with her husband's infidelities, which made her feel abandoned.

Dr. Masterson: Notice how identifying the precipitation stress helps to organize the clinical material.

Participant: In her Irish family of origin, Mrs. B. was supposed to be the nice one. She was very pretty, though now she's overweight. She's a bleached blonde, very Felliniesque, with this incredible laugh. She still considers herself attractive to men. Her sister was more privileged. Her brother was close to her until he married.

In the last two sessions, Mrs. B. fondly remembered a photograph of herself, holding her father's hand when she was four. The picture was given away by her brother to one of his girlfriends. Mrs. B. sees this as an irretrievable loss and betrayal. Now her brother won't speak to her.

Her mother and sister live together in the city and her father is dead. Her father was alcoholic. Mother and her own sister were twins and often switched roles when Dad was courting Mrs. B's mother. She now sees this as evidence of poor boundaries.

As treatment went on, B. revealed that family sexual boundaries were weak. She believes her mother took her father away from her.

Now, I'm going to describe a pattern that seems significant. Mrs. B. sees her sister as a threat to her marriage and thinks her husband had sex with her. She thinks her mother takes her husband away from her when he spends nights at her house unexpectedly and fails to come home. Because he's a construction worker in the city, he sometimes doesn't go home on Wednesdays. Mom colludes with Mrs. B.'s sister and allows her to drink with J., Mrs. B.'s husband.

In J.'s family of origin, boundaries were also weak. J. and his mother are said to have watched together a woman undress across the way. This is a recurrent story. J. had an affair with his own brother's wife. Mrs. B's mother-in-law made no objection.

Dr. Masterson: Are you sure this isn't a television soap opera? The question here is not diagnosis, but who was doing what with whom.

Participant: The mother-in-law apparently said to her, "What do you expect?" When she first met her, the mother-in-law said she didn't like Mrs. B. because she had blue eyes and you can't trust people with blue eyes.

Dr. Masterson: I'm beginning to feel overwhelmed because the real question here is why she puts up with all this.

Participant: She's afraid that he'll leave her. If he leaves her, she falls apart.

Dr. Masterson: Did you convey this to her?

Participant: Yes. I did say, "I'm not going to ask you to leave him, it's up to you what you decide to do. But why are you putting up with all this stuff?"

Dr. Masterson: It would have been worthwhile to explore what happened in the other treatment. Maybe the therapist didn't ask her to leave him. Maybe the therapist said, "Why do you stay with him?" He's trying to confront her compliance with all this self-destructive behavior. This kind of situation automatically makes you wonder if she was sexually abused too. Is she having affairs on the side when she drinks?

Participant: She got involved in some form of threesome because of her husband and alcohol, and she feels terrible shame. She recalls this story every once in a while. She did this only once.

Dr. Masterson: What is it that impels you to present the case?

Participant: It's because I don't know what to do with her.

Dr. Masterson: Tell us the process now—what she did, what you did about it, and what confuses you.

Participant: She started by saying that she thought I thought she was stupid and that I disapproved of her because she's alcoholic. All of a sudden, I saw this linkage between all the women in her life who are linked to each other in some kind of pattern to separate her from her husband. I felt I had to confront her on every example of this behavior.

For example, she believed I thought she was stupid. She went on, then, to explain that it was her mother who was responsible for her being held back in First Grade. She was never given opportunities, she was disadvantaged, especially intellectually. I had to stop her and say, "You're saying this about me, but it's really your mother. Do you see that?" She said, "But I love my mother. She took my father away from me." Do you think she's borderline?

Dr. Masterson: It sounds like it . . . unless she could be what we sometimes call inadequate psychopath. A psychopathic personality. We now call it antisocial, which is a very bad term. For instance, many of them are not antisocial. There's the inadequate psychopath who doesn't feel very much and goes from acting out to acting out to acting out. But I think she's probably borderline.

Participant: She also cried a lot in this session.

Dr. Masterson: What is it that confuses you in dealing with her?

Participant: I'm confused because she keeps bringing up something like the mother, and then it's another friend who's triangulated her, and it goes on and on. Is it enough to confront each, single thing? And then is she ever going to grow? Is she ever going to, because she falls apart?

Dr. Masterson: How does she fall apart?

Participant: One of the precipitants of her falling apart, oddly enough, was that her son's girlfriend left him and she was so agitated that she started to skip from subject to subject.

Her best friend betrayed her, I think she's stupid, or else I disapprove of her.

Dr. Masterson: You don't think she's schizophrenic. But that's not falling apart. She's upset, right?

Participant: Very. What I said was incorrect because there is regression and disintegration, when Mrs. B.'s husband doesn't come home. That's another thing. Mrs. B. becomes confused, cries, and complains of being fragmented, of "falling apart."

Dr. Masterson: What does that mean?

Participant: I was seen as rejecting, skipping from one subject to another.

Dr. Masterson: I think there are two reasons you're having trouble. One is she is presenting you with such a variety of acting-out and everybody is acting out and everybody else is acting out on their acting out, so it's as if you've got this circus going on all the time and you're trying to figure out what you are looking at now. Is this the clown? The juggler? The high-flying trapeze artist?

You end up focusing on *what* rather than *why*. That's the first part of the dilemma. The second is that you are put off by, and made anxious by, her distress because of the terms you use: "She is falling apart, she's disintegrating." You are identifying with the projections she is sending you. And what is she doing? In my vocabulary, when she doesn't have her rewarding unit defense, she acts out helplessness, which is not falling apart. It's, "I can't do anything about myself. Somebody else has got to."

Participant: Makes me focus?

Dr. Masterson: Right. You're feeling it—she also projects her helplessness into you.

Participant: And then I think it's terrific that she hasn't said she wasn't coming back, because all the way through this she would say I may not come back.

Dr. Masterson: And what do you say to that?

Participant: What do I say to that? "I hope you do, it's up to you."

Dr. Masterson: You don't hope she does.

Participant: No, I don't.

Dr. Masterson: She's very attractive?

Participant: Yes.

Dr. Masterson: She knows how it use it.

Participant: She knows she's charming.

Dr. Masterson: You don't hope she comes back. You don't care whether she comes back or not. This is not your life, it's her life. You're not going to come back? You sit here and you talk about all this trouble and you tell me you're not going to come back? What kind of a perspective is that on yourself?

How can you plumb this myriad of acting-out? They all have a commonality which applies in general with dealing with borderlines who do not activate and support themselves. You find a central dimension that applies to everything they do, whether it's their work, relationship with their children, relationship with a spouse, relationship with peers. The pathologic ego operates in fantasy, not in reality. So her fantasy is she's got to not manage herself and then her alcoholic husband and all this coterie of people will take care of her. So she has to be helpless. However, if she does manage herself, it will all disappear.

Knowing that, whatever she's talking about: the mother, the sister, etc., you constantly intervene with: "Why do you put up with this? Why do you not support yourself? Why do you let yourself be treated this way? It's no wonder you're drinking, with what you have to contend with. I think rather than contend with it you turn to the alcohol." In addition, she is doing the same with you, the therapist. She's not coming in and working on her problem. You are to take care of her.

Participant: I just remembered, in my terror at standing here, I forgot why she didn't really fall apart. On the weekend her husband told her that a co-worker had been knocked off this huge building by a beam. She said, "I've been saying all these terrible things about him in group. I haven't been good enough to him. He went to Vietnam and came back and all I do is criticize him. Why don't I put up with it? I'm going to leave treatment." That's what it was.

Dr. Masterson: That's where you have to confront her.

Participant: I had taken this seriously as a disintegration, but it really was a regression.

Dr. Masterson: But, remember, she operates through projection and we all have a tendency to identify with projections. She's playing you like a piano. And for what purpose? In order not to feel and look at what her problem is inside her head.

Participant: I could say, "Why do you put up with this?"

Dr. Masterson: No. She says, "My husband told me somebody fell off the roof and, my God, I had attacked him and he went to Vietnam." What could you say to her?

Participant: I don't know.

Dr. Masterson: All right. Anybody else?

Audience: What relevance is that to you?

Dr. Masterson: Right. What does the one have to do with the other? What it has to do with the other, I suspect, is that she's frightened of being abandoned by her husband and this co-worker dies and this reinforces her fear of being abandoned by her husband. He may abandon her because she criticized him. This is a fantasy which she thinks is a reality. You have to constantly confront that. Why do you make so much of this? How long have they been married? Since 1967?

One of the nice things about working with a borderline is you can use a sense of humor, but with a narcissistic disorder nothing is funny. Humor helps the borderline to get some distance from his pain, soothes it a bit, and it reinforces the observing ego.

I might say something like, "I know you're afraid of his leaving you, but it's a puzzle to me why?" This is getting her attention. "What do you mean?" "Well, it seems to me he likes alcohol better than you, so why would he bother to leave you as long as he's got the alcohol?"

That sounds like a terrible thing to say. And it would be a terrible thing to say if you were not confronting acting-out.

Another example was a borderline woman in her 40s, working at a level below her capacity but making quite a bit of money. Her intimate relations were as follows: She'd get a postcard from Johannesburg from this friend who is going to be in New York next week. The man would appear and they'd have a terrific five days—drinking, going to shows, making love. He was in love with her; then he'd disappear. The next postcard came from another man from London and the same sequence was repeated. After three or four of these, I began to raise questions. You don't go for the jugular with your confrontations; you start at the periphery and you work in.

Finally, one day I said to her: "There is something I don't understand here and maybe you can clarify it for me.

It seems to me that in order to qualify for your bed, a man has to come by plane. Why is that?" She got the message which she integrated. And she stopped the plane business and guess what happened. A man appeared on the scene in New York and she dissolved with anxiety. The distancing defense was gone. There was now a possibility of continuity, against which the distancing had been a defense.

So if you can get a metaphor which has some humor to it, it helps.

Participant: What would you do if a patient then says you're right, but I can't? This happened to me last night.

Dr. Masterson: One of the nice things about this work is that there are a variety of things you can do. Remember that silence itself is a confrontation. You are saying to the patient, the ball is in your court, do with it whatever you want. So the first thing you could do is say nothing and see what happens.

Participant: Would you let the session just end?

Dr. Masterson: These are all judgment calls with each situation. I might. I have done that and I've done it over a series of sessions. I would say to this patient—I don't know whether it applies here, but where it does apply: "You are on a sitdown strike, I mean that you're managing your anger by sitting there and not budging until I speak for you. That isn't going to happen." And from that point on I don't say a word. I might sit through the whole next session as well and at the end I might say, "Well, I see you are still doing it."

The other option would be to explore. The bottom line would be, "I don't understand what you're doing here. If you don't want to look into this, what are you doing here?" Don't be afraid to bring that up. So many therapists are afraid to bring that up.

Question: I did bring that up and he said yes . . .

Dr. Masterson: Then he should stop. I would say to him, "Obviously, we see this differently and the decision is up to you. If you want to stop, fine." Make sure that you oppose his point of view because he might come back again, he still might be testing.

I don't worry about patients staying in treatment. I worry about whether or not I did the job right. If I do the job right, I can't control their staying or leaving. I've rarely had a patient leave who then did treatment with someone else. They stop because they don't want treatment. Everybody who comes into your office doesn't want treatment. They want a whole variety of things, but not necessarily treatment. I have told patients, "You don't want treatment. You're doing this to arrange something with your family or your husband or your wife. It has nothing to do with treatment." If you don't do that, you're colluding with the patient's resistance.

A borderline woman came to see me, with a tremendous problem with her father and her mother. She acted out sexually and had the strangest collection of men. I confronted her about all that and she responded by getting rid of these men. Finally she married. She found a man who wanted to be a daddy, as opposed to a husband. He just takes care of her, overindulges and infantilizes her, and doesn't require her to be responsible for herself. She stops treatment, of course. Who needs treatment? She's gotten what she wanted. As a matter of fact, she married him at the point in treatment when we had gotten through all the other men and she was just about to start the internal investigation of the problem with the father. So she had acted out as a defense, which I pointed out at the time, but she wantd to do it anyway.

Two years later she wants to see me again. What's the problem? "I want to have a baby and my husband said to me that he already has to take care of one baby and he doesn't want another." He frustrated her. What did she do? She started an affair with another man, who, unfortunately, falls in love with her. He wants her to leave husband/daddy. That's when she calls me, because she's stuck. But she doesn't want treatment. She wants me somehow to work that situation out.

I told her the reason she came to me was the same reason she started the affair. She couldn't handle the situation with her husband about not having the baby. I said I didn't think she was any more prepared to deal with it with me now than she had been before. Thus, I didn't see any point in treatment.

Incidentally, her husband had connections with the Mafia. I said, "If I were you, I'd be very careful about this affair because if he finds out it may go very badly without your being able to protect yourself. She hasn't come back.

Participant: People sometimes stop treatment and come back later. I've had two patients who have come back and another patient who has left the second time, I don't know if she's coming back or not. But it takes some confidence to deal with it.

Dr. Masterson: Inside yourself. Of course it does.

Participant: Another way of turning things around is to suddenly decide, at termination, to start to work.

Dr. Masterson: In other words, you could say to the patient that he's not getting anywhere and if he doesn't make progress by such and such a date, there's no point in continuing.

Participant: I wouldn't say it that way. I would say that I think we've reached a level where we're not making the sort of headway that I feel you need, so we're going to set a termination date. It's not a panacea, but there are times when it's helpful.

Dr. Masterson: Don't use the word *we*. It's a bad word. It should be *you, you, you*. It isn't *we*. The patient wants it to be *we*.

Question: Is there a shorter term approach to the borderline patient?

Dr. Masterson: Absolutely. The whole first case presented yesterday was for that purpose. That patient was seen once a week. The first half of *Psychotherapy of the Borderline Adult* is about what I call confrontive therapy, where the patient is seen once a week. It's extremely effective because patients respond to confrontation. Their work improves, their relationships improve. You don't have to put the patient on the couch three and four times a week, even with higher-level borderline. The higher-level patients benefit, too, from confrontive therapy.

Participant: But I thought you had said you didn't think people could work through.

Dr. Masterson: No, they don't work through. Let's define what we're talking about. When I talk about intensive analytic treatment and working through the abandonment depression, that's the ultimate goal of treatment. You get rid of the anchor on the abandonment depression, you get rid of the anchor on development, the self emerges, the patient goes through the oedipal phase, and he or she becomes a healthy person, or close to it. This is what analytic treatment is all about. Vulnerability to separation stress is removed. There is what I call the flowering of individuation. The patient becomes what seems like a new person. It's not new, but all those capacities they had kept in the closet because of anxiety and depression start to emerge. That's analytic treatment, which takes three times a week over a long period of time. It's well worth the effort because the results are so great.

In confrontive therapy, the patient is seen once a week. The goal is ego repair. All of those primitive mechanisms of defense, the defects in ego functioning—denial, avoidance, projection—operate at the cost of reality perception. What you mainly do in treatment is confrontation. The patients take it in and heal those holes in their ego. Now they see reality as it is. Basically, what they do is strip their rewarding/withdrawing unit projections from reality and deal with reality on its own terms. Work improves, relationships improve. They have a new life. They still have the developmental arrest and, underneath, they still have the abandonment depression.

By the way, in this shorter-term treatment, you should avoid those therapeutic activities that draw the patient into a deeper relationship—transference, fantasies, dreams, and memories.

The reason you avoid them is that you don't want to draw the patient deeper into the relationship, because you're not intending to work it through. Now, that doesn't mean you don't let them talk about these matters. But, unlike analytic therapy where you would take those up systematically to investigate, with the investigation actually becoming the principal vehicle as you get into the working-through phase, you don't do that in confrontive therapy. You let the patient talk, but you don't take it up for investigation.

In addition, the patient has to find some more adaptive ways to deal with episodes of separation stress, which produce abandonment depression. For example, an alcoholic could take up jogging or tennis or playing chess, an activity that holds them and contains affect.

One of my patients described it this way: "It's like being in the ocean with your feet on the bottom and you see a swell coming and you have to learn how to tread water until the swell passes." If the swell doesn't pass, they'll then regress, become symptomatic, and come back for treatment.

When a borderline is exposed to too much separation

stress, he or she loses previously learned insight. That's the only way they can activate those old defenses. When that happens, they'll come back to treatment. But you haven't lost previously learned insight and what it took you six months to accomplish the first time around, you can do in a matter of weeks.

The point I want to make is that confrontive therapy is extremely effective. The other side of the coin is the narcissistic disorder. In general, with a narcissistic disorder, the more you see the patient, the better. Once-a-week treatment with a narcissistic disorder is slow going. Since they don't respond to confrontation, what you can achieve is limited compared to what you can achieve with a borderline. But it doesn't mean that in certain cases you can't do a lot.

For example, a 64-year-old man who was an outstanding business success displayed a classic exhibitionistic narcissistic disorder. He had severe depression and panic after the break-up of a relationship and the onset of angina. He has had two marriages and a long history of sexual acting-out with women. Then he gives me his history. Between ages two and seven he had severe illnesses, was bedridden, and was expected to die. The way he dealt with his feelings was to erect this grandiose fantasy role that he was able to translate into reality.

The way he had dealt with his fear of death was with a narcissistic defense. Aging, signified by the angina, was overcoming this role-playing defense. Over a number of sessions I finally made the interpretation to him that angina and getting older had brought back what he thought he had put away, which was his fear of death. And this is what was driving him crazy. There was a huge difference between his symptom and the prospect of dying.

He experienced dramatic relief, like one sees in the movies. He had had five years of analysis and the analyst never said anything. He couldn't understand why I talked.

It's as if he's had a magical experience and he cannot believe it.

I think what he's saying is he can't believe he's going to live, he's not going to die, and somehow it has something to do with the treatment.

In general, the rule of thumb is it's a lot harder to treat a narcissistic disorder once a week. Also, the older they are, the better. When younger, they think they're going to be able to be perfect and admired. When they get older, they've been bounced around by life so that the idea is beginning to occur that maybe they're not going to make it to being perfect and admired.

Participant: I'm having some problem negotiating with a high-level borderline who had come into treatment with a depression and with a great deal of clarity about what had happened, but also acting out a lot.

Dr. Masterson: How often are you seeing the patient?

Participant: Once a week.

Dr. Masterson: Then there's no question. Why aren't you confronting the acting-out?

Participant: I am confronting the acting-out.

Dr. Masterson: What is she doing?

Participant: Occasionally not getting up to leave the office at the end of the interview, which is recurrent.

Dr. Masterson: What do you do about that?

Participant: Basically, the most effective thing I do is to say, "This is harmful to you." And she tends to back out a little bit.

Dr. Masterson: Forget the hurting you. Remember that there is a conflict between acting out and insight. When somebody is acting out, they're not available for insight. Did you try just saying, "The session is over. Why are you still here?"

Participant: She'd say, "I can't go, it's too painful."

Dr. Masterson: You might also say, "This is part of the problem you have, not only here but outside here. You must start to learn to control it right here, right now. Good-bye." I had a lot worse problem than that. I finally said to this patient, "If you don't leave the office this instant, I will call the police." These statements are all underlining reality. It's interesting that you are caught the way she is caught. She is in the abandonment depression. That's okay, but she's also acting out and she has manipulated you into the position that somehow you have to do something about her abandonment depression that interferes with confronting her acting-out. You want to hone in on what she was feeling before she acted out. Why couldn't she hold on to the feeling?

When a patient reports falling apart, you want to get a detailed description of what went on before that occurred. "What were you feeling? What was happening? What efforts did you make to manage it? What did you think to do?"

When borderline patients experience pain, they become helpless. They don't think of things to do. They don't even think that that's the idea. You confront that, getting across to them that when people are upset, they usually find some way of handling it or soothing it, rather than exaggerating it.

You're ambivalent with your patient. You haven't given her the message that she has no choice. You're still giving a little too much leeway to her defensiveness. You might say, "I don't understand when you're so smart and this is so clear why you keep playing footsie with this problem and with me?" Also, you better figure out yourself some way of dealing with her not leaving the session. That has to stop!

Remember that the most effective defense is the transference acted-out defense. Patients who are late for sessions and patients who may not leave must be dealt with because these acts interfere with the momentum. You constantly have to talk to her about working at cross purposes with herself. You say, "There is no point in your feeling all this pain and then not getting up and leaving my office. Do you want to do it or don't you? It seems to me you have the capacity to do it and you've worked very hard to get to this point." She's testing if you think she can do it. Patients have such lack of confidence that they can do it that they have to know whether you do. So they keep pushing you and pushing you.

Dr. Nagel's case was a beautiful example of that. Every time she confronted her, she found another way to test. "Do you really mean this?" And you have to, of course, say, "Yes, I do." That's what the work is about.

Question: What happens if a parent dies during the treatment?

Dr. Masterson: That's very tough. If it's a father or a mother whom they have lived with, what will happen is that the momentum of the working through will stop and first they must mourn the present reality relationship with the parent. If it's done effectively, this will then lead back to the abandonment depression.

What you have to do as a therapist is back off from interpretations at the deeper abandonment depression level and come back and deal with this situation in the here and now and give them space in order to mourn it, if they can. If they can't, which they may well not, then you have to deal with that. You must confront that so they can get back in touch with it. That's a very complicated thing in a patient in treatment at that stage.

Question: How do you handle a countertransference evoked mostly by the patient's behavior?

Dr. Masterson: There are many ways. If it has caused you to act in ways that are not therapeutic, then you have to acknowledge that you blew it. You can use it as what we call a signal anxiety or litmus test. You look back at what the patient is doing to produce your feeling and you interpret it. If it hasn't gotten into the action and the work, you don't have to acknowledge it to the patient. If it has, you have to. You may even acknowledge it if it hasn't, if you think it's important enough.

Question: Can you use your countertransference to make a diagnosis?

Dr. Masterson: I don't think the way to go about diagnosis is through your countertransference feelings. They should certainly be secondary phenomena, not that it's not relevant. I think you should make your diagnosis on the observable objective evidence, as demonstrated in the history and the patient's behavior with you.

I know there are some people, like Searles, who use their so-called countertransference fairly well. I think he's very intuitive about it and he gets away with it. Maybe, if you're terribly healthy, you might get away with it. If you're not, you will be in trouble. So I would use the countertransference as additional confirming data.

I'll give you an example. This was an anorexic patient who was borderline and had been treated in the hospital. On discharge she was referred to me because her therapist went into the Navy. She had had a very good relationship with him and she had done well. I think, in retrospect, that she was moving from a pre-oedipal to an oedipal kind of transference.

She started with me three times a week. And for months all I got from her was anger. Not at her other therapist who had left, but at me and my inadequacies. After a while, I got pretty fed up with this and recognized that I was fed up with it, that I was identifying with her projection of how bad I was. Then I started to investigate the relationship of her anger to the loss of the other therapist.

But the key to it was not that. Rather, in her relationship with her mother, her mother had used *her* as a mother. So she was the target of all the mother's anger and depression. The mother used to sit and do with her what she was doing with me. Her way of dealing with the rage and depression at losing the therapist was to put me in the role of herself and to play out the role of the mother with me and thereby externalize the abandonment depression. It wasn't until we got around that that she could get back to work it through.

Participant: What is the Masterson position on working with addictions?

Dr. Masterson: Addictions can go beyond psychodynamics. Some alcoholic addictions are biochemical, which may be true of other addictions, too. There may be some biological factors involved. But where the psychodynamic factors are part of it, our point of view is that it's a defense.

Participant: You don't send the person to take care of the addiction while working it through?

Dr. Masterson: Oh, absolutely. Doesn't everyone agree that you do not do psychotherapy with anyone on drugs or alcohol? They go to AA, they go to a drug rehab, and they stick it out. If they go back to sustained drinking or drugs, you stop the treatment.

Our basic position is that treatment and addiction compete with each other. There are two ways to deal with your problems. You can allow yourself to feel them and work on them or you can drown them with alcohol or drugs.

Participant: What about patients who come to me because they're stuck with their therapists and often on a lot of medication?

Dr. Masterson: One of the troubles with medications is that we have so many of them and they're so good that they can be used for countertransferential purposes.

Participant: What about patients who haven't responded normally to medication?

Dr. Masterson: We see a lot of these patients. The first thing we do is take them off the drugs in order to do a basic reevaluation. Medication can have a lot of side effects that cloud the clinical picture.

Participant: Your stance is a correct one, but not everybody agrees. There are plenty of psychiatrists who put the patients on the couch and try to analyze them.

Question: What about projective identification where the patient takes you down to where you're as bad as he is? He has you stuck against the wall at that point. Where are you then?

Dr. Masterson: When you get to that level, you're in bad shape. You have lost the ball game. You have to go and see somebody for supervision, get some distance, or transfer the patient. Can you be more specific?

Question: "Your therapy is helping me. You're the big doctor, but you haven't done anything for me. When are you going to start helping me?"

Dr. Masterson: "How can you say that after spending weeks here ignoring and avoiding all my comments? Now you want to accuse me of not helping you? It's you who are not willing to help yourself."

I had an example of what you're talking about that shocked me. It shouldn't have, I should have known better, but it still did. A therapist had this patient on the couch. The patient's father didn't want to have anything to do with him, so he bought him off by giving him a lot of money and ignoring him. The patient lived on the money, did not work, and was on heroin. Clearly, the patient wasn't getting anywhere and he complained to the therapist. What was the therapist doing? He was making interpretations and, for some strange reason, they didn't work. The therapist was saying, in effect, "It's not me, it's you. I'm making these fancy interpretations that can't be wrong."

They get a consultant—from the same group. What does the consultant say to the patient? That it's not the therapist's fault, it's the patient's fault. He is on heroin, and not working, his father is treating him like a two-year-old, and none of this was dealt with. Yet the consultant says, "It's not your therapist, it's you."

The patient was "threatening" to leave, so the therapist asked me to see the patient for a consultation. I have a technique I call therapeutic astonishment. It's a very useful form of confrontation. In the first session I said, "I'm astonished at what you're telling me here." He replied, "Oh, yeah, why?" "Well, you're 29 years old, you're not even working, and you're taking heroin. We'll have to talk more about that next time." I was confronting his defenses to see what he could manage.

In the next session, I told him my view was very different from that of the other consultant. My view was that he was not in a situation to take advantage of treatment, regardless of what his therapist did. "You're not supporting yourself with work, you're drowning your emotions in heroin. I don't know whether what your therapist was doing was right or wrong, but it surely was not going to help until you get a job and give up heroin." Then, if the therapist knows what he's doing, the patient would get someplace.

I called the therapist and told him his behavior ended

up being a repetition of the father's. The therapist was neglecting his treatment needs just as the father had neglected his emotional needs. I said, "You've got to confront his avoidance of responsibility for himself, tell him you won't treat him if he stays on heroin, and he's got to get a job, he's got to pay for his treatment. In addition, get him off the couch, put him in the chair, and talk about how he manages."

About five months later, the therapist called me back. "I can't believe it," he said. "You should see the change. It's absolutely magic. He went off the heroin, he got a job, he's depressed but managing everything, and the treatment is off the ground."

Participant: Let's go back to the scenario where you tell him to get a job. He says, "I don't want a job. I don't want to work like my father did. I'm okay. I go out to the golf course and I don't have enough money to play golf, but I'm just hitting the ball and maybe some day somebody will pay for me so I can play. And you know, I'm not going to do what you tell me."

Dr. Masterson: "It's up to you to do whatever you want to do. But I think your perspective is all wrong. You're telling me you're okay, but you're on heroin. I have yet to meet anyone on heroin who is okay."

Participant: I've spelled it out: "If you want me to help you, you're going to have to work in here, set up the boundaries, the whole deal." I told him, "You're not interested in working," and I told the family also.

Dr. Masterson: Well there are people who don't want to do it.

Participant: Was there something else I could have done?

Dr. Masterson: No, as long as you confronted him.

Participant: He was saying, "There's nothing wrong with me. I don't belong here."

Dr. Masterson: If you feel a patient is going to leave, I consider that a therapeutic emergency. Then I will throw out things I wouldn't ordinarily, bounce back and forth between confrontations and interpretations. "You think you're okay. I think you're okay because you're afraid to take a chance on yourself."

Participant: I've done that. The only problem there is the question of suicide.

Dr. Masterson: Sure, this could all be a protection against suicidal drive.

Participant: When you recommend that somebody go into chemical preventive treatment and they do that, do you wait a period of time before starting psychotherapy?

Dr. Masterson: I'll tell him to go to a rehab and get off the drugs. If an alcoholic comes in, if he won't go to rehab, I won't treat him. He has to go to AA.

Participant: Is there a period of sobriety?

Dr. Masterson: It depends on how bad it is. I might try a little to confront them and point out what they're doing to themselves, but not for all that long. Their denial is so monumental. I think you should take them for consultation and then you tell them what has to be done. If they want to do it, they'll do it.

Question: Could you relate confrontations to normal separation? Is it corrective?

Dr. Masterson: It's a corrective against the defenses that prevent separation individuation. In other words, what you're confronting is what's keeping the patient from individuating. If you're successful, then the individuation takes over. The normal mother does this. She wants her child to grow up. She takes pleasure in his growth. So, as the child grows, he gets positive responses. As he regresses and avoids, he gets some sort of confrontation from the mother: "Don't stay in the house all day. Why aren't you out playing with your friends?"

10

Workshop

Peter E. Sifneos, M.D.

Dr. Sifneos: We now have an opportunity to discuss brief psychotherapy a little more. I'm particularly interested in questions that you may have.

But let me first give you a brief overview of its development, starting with the point made yesterday that the original cases of Freud and of some of the early analysts were of short-term duration. Referring to the case of Dora, that celebrated case of hysteria that Freud had, he treated her over a period of about eight months. There is a footnote in terms of the follow-up that she had done quite well and had given up her father for now, establishing meaningful relationships with men. Freud did not think that follow-up work at the time was neccessary, but it's nice that he made that point.

In addition, there is the celebrated case of short-term psychotherapy in child psychiatry with little Hans, the little boy who had the phobia of horses. Freud treated him by means of his father and there we have, again, accidentally, an 18- or 19-year follow-up. He was now a young man and Freud saw him and asked him whether he remembered anything or whether he had any phobias. The answer was no, he was feeling fine.

There were, also, at least anecdotally speaking, some short-term cases while Freud was on his vacation in the Alps or elsewhere. Various people would join him and they would have some conversation on whatever the problem was. There were some eminent people such as Gustav Mahler, for instance, who had sexual problems and problems of composing. Thereafter, he became very prolific.

So there were these very short-term interventions. I shall come to that point because we have also seen some patients for an evaluation interview only. Then, after a while, particularly since we had this research where patients had to wait to be controlled, we discovered that at the end of about five or six months, when the patient was ready to start therapy, the therapist would say the problems had been resolved. What do you mean the problems had been resolved? Well, during this waiting period, the patient says, and there are some very interesting examples, that he or she had somehow or other gained a momentum from that first evaluation interview. From then on, things started moving along in terms of the patient's own ability to resolve the problems.

We are particularly interested in these patients as to the nature of the psychological structure and what it is that one intervention set in motion. Let me give you an example.

This was a young woman who was very anxious, particularly about her relationship with her father, which was a constant battle. This had started about when she was 14. On one occasion, her mother was away visiting her own mother and she woke up in the middle of the night and there was her father, who was drunk, caressing her breasts. She felt horrified, as well as kind of excited. From then on, this relationship with her father had gone from bad to worse. She was living at home and there were constant fights. This is what prompted her to get psychotherapy—because she could not, in a sense, relate to anybody in this country.

But the interesting thing was that she had gone to Europe on two occasions and had relationships there. Once she was even thinking of getting married to a young man in Ireland. When she returned to the states, her father discouraged her and she gave up that relationship, as well as a similar one the following year.

She was seen by one of our social workers for an evaluation interview. Usually, under this intake system, therapists see their own patients and then we in the professional team get together. The person who has evaluated the patient presents the case and we have a discussion. The patient comes in, is interviewed by one of us, and we hope to give a recommendation to the patient that particular day.

The social worker who saw her first asked the patient if she had ever thought of the possibility that the reason her father was so nasty to her was that he wanted to stop himself from repeating this humiliating experience with her. That stopped her. She hadn't thought of this possibility, but saw him only as a nasty person. Thus her anger at him.

She came to our intake and the same problem was presented. When we heard that she was having a relationship every year in Europe and no relationships in this country, one of the members of the team asked, "Has it occurred to you that perhaps the only reason you don't have relationships with American men is because your father is here. What a difference the Atlantic Ocean makes! You can cross it and have such good relationships over there."

Again, that brought her up short, but that was it. She was put on our waiting list because she was a control patient; we thought she fulfilled the criteria. When the therapist who was assigned to her five months later saw her, she said, "There's no problem." You remember, I mentioned that we put down criteria for outcome. Criteria for outcome were of course, that she would have some kind of relationship in this country, that the relationship with her father would have improved, and there wouldn't be this constant battle. Essentially, she would be symptom-free. Well, she fulfilled these criteria.

So he said, "What is there to treat?" She told him that she had moved out of the house, she had reestablished a relationship with her father that was not an ambivalent back-and-forth situation, and she was symptom-free.

That one interview with these two interventions set in motion, in a fairly healthy individual, the possibility of doing that work for herself. So, coming back to these cases of Freud, it is possible that what he was doing with Mahler and many other famous people was something of this kind and that these people were, as we call them, "right" for this kind of intervention.

Many of you may remember from your college days quantitative analysis in chemistry, where you draw acid drop by drop and suddenly that last drop changes the solution. It all becomes pink because it becomes base.

Well, it's something like that. We have that last drop, that intervention, in a person who is ripe to deal with her own actions and has that ego capacity that can set things in motion. I shall come to that point because it is of interest in terms of follow-up of our work.

Going back to the historical development, I mentioned yesterday some of the efforts of Ferenczi and Rank in introducing these kinds of behavioral techniques. Rank was interesting, also, because he had an obsession that all psychological difficulties with each and every one of us have to do with a birth trauma and he proceeded to recommend that all psychoanalysis should last exactly nine months in order to balance things with gestation. That was not very enthusiastically received; he was asked to leave the International Psycho Analytic Association.

Ferenczi said that his active interpretations that rewarded and reinforced the patient were aimed particularly at shortening psychoanalysis because by 1915 or 1916 it had become long-term. I think that had something to do with the enthusiasm of the early analysts who changed from a kind of Kraepelinian rigidity, like DSM-III-R that we have returned to, to acceptance of the dymanic fluidity of the human mind. Their enthusiasm led them to put everybody on the couch. Of course, some patients were not capable of dealing with this. As you all know, if you put a schizophrenic patient on the couch, within about two minutes it's Pandora's box. Those people who have good ego strength take a long period of time to allow themselves to free associate, because it is such a difficult thing to describe your most intimate thoughts with somebody listening.

Even Freud, as you know, wrote a paper in 1937 on analysis terminable and interminable. There are several reasons why Freud mentioned that analysis might be interminable. One is trauma, which we have rediscovered now, but as if nobody else had known about it. The other was a rigidity of defenses to such a degree that they would be impossible to penetrate. And the third and very interesting one, at least when I was at the Boston Psychoanalytic Institute, was that the analyst's personality problems may interfere with this particular situation. Well, we don't like to talk about those things. Analysts don't have personality problems.

Anyway, that might lead to the interminable analysis. This situation continued up to the exodus of the analysts from Austria and Germany in the late 30s. Then World War II arrived, bringing the utilization of dynamic interventions to help the Armed Services people who had difficulties. Rather that being sent from the Pacific or from Europe, they could be helped over there and quickly returned to active duty. There was an enormous amount of interest in psychodynamic interventions. When the veterans returned after the war, there was an enormous amount of interest in the late 40s and 50s, lasting, I would say, up to about the mid-1960s. I would say that in the 50s there was no chairperson of any Department of Psychiatry in a university in this country who was not analytically trained or an analyst. The whole thing has changed since then. There are reasons for that and we might return to that discussion.

Very briefly, it was then that Franz Alexander in Chicago was doing work on creating a corrective emotional experience. This involved the ability of the therapist, with expectations on the part of the patient, to somehow repeat the problem that the patient may have had, for example, with a person in authority—a young man who has had difficulties with his father and difficulties with men in authority and his bosses, and comes in because he has lost his job two or three times.

When this young man sees a male therapist, you might expect in the transference that he would have the same kind of anxiety about the relationship that he would have with someone in authority. Alexander's point was that if the therapist acted in a kind of active, benign, supportive way, he would alter at least some of the expectations and everybody in authority would be seen that way. This was called a corrective emotional experience, as Alexander wrote in his book, *Psychoanalytic Psychotherapy*, in 1946. Ernest Jones, the biographer of Freud, was asked to review the book and refused because he saw no point in an analyst reviewing a book that doesn't use the word "unconscious."

The book does use the word "unconscious" six or seven times, so it's clear that Jones didn't open the book. He didn't care because the so-called manipulation of the transference—that is, acting in a benign way to undo certain expectations—was considered to be taboo and contrary to the neutrality of the analyst.

Some people talk about the neutrality of the analyst even though Freud was showing patients his books and artifacts, recommending coffee shops to go to for good cakes in Vienna, etc. Very neutral, indeed!

As a result of this emormous interest in psychodynamic interventions, the situation became such that the only way to deal with the demand was to set up the infamous waiting list.

In 1954, I was a candidate in training at Boston Psycho Analytic Society and I had to wait for two and a half years for my training analyst. I was told that I was very lucky because there were some who had to wait four years. All the clinics were jammed and there were long waiting lists. Indeed, there were not enough therapists. In those days, the only therapy available was long-term psychoanalytic psychotherapy for borderline and narcissistic patients (of course, those terms were not used at the time), electric shock and insulin shock for the psychoses, and that was it. Chlorpromazine didn't appear until 1955.

So, the only way to deal with this issue was to put patients on the waiting list. And this prompted the London study saying that those who get psychotherapy and those who don't do just as well. It also said there wasn't a single paper demonstrating the efficacy of psychotherapy.

The first point is not correct because there are patients we cannot help by psychotherapy, but there are also some we can. But the second point was true. There wasn't a single attempt to look, in a more systematic way, into the efficacy of psychotherapy so as to be able to demonstrate it on a scientific research basis. Results were all on an anecdotal basis. This is the reason why I emphasize the importance of videotape, but we can come to that later on.

Meanwhile, at the Massachusetts General Hospital I was asked to fill in as director of the Psychiatric Clinic for a few months. I accepted the job and then discovered there were at least 200 people on the waiting list for long-term psychotherapy.

We wondered then if we could do what we had done at Wellesley, this time in a clinical situation, in a hospital psychiatric clinic. It was then that we decided to set up the intake conferences which I have described to you. A patient would be seen, evaluated, and then brought to a group. Usually, it was an interdisciplinary group of 10 or 12 people, mostly psychiatrists, psychologists, social workers, and students in these specialties. Occasionally, we also had some social scientists.

We had five teams, one for each day of the week. All patients that came to the clinic that particular day were to be evaluated by the team and, if possible, at the end of the day given a recommendation as to whether they should be referred privately, get long-term psychotherapy, or whatever. It was at that time that we saw the patient whom I described earlier (see pages 79–80), the man with phobias who was soon to be married. We were able, then, to treat him successfully over a short period of time.

Thus, we decided that it was of interest to see those patients. I told you about seeing 50 at first and interviewing 21 of those 50 in follow-up about a year and a half to two years later. We found that they had talked about how much they had learned about themselves. The word "learning" was emphasized.

What was striking was what these patients said about their improvement in relationships with key people that had disturbed them previously. Their symptomatic improvement was better, but not complete. That is, some of them said, "I used to be very anxious, but I'm less anxious now. The anxiety interfered in such and such a way and now it doesn't interfere."

We decided then to change the criteria for selection. Now the first criterion for selection, as I mentioned to you yesterday, was a circumscribed chief difficulty. Not so much what the patient emphasizes, but what we think is the basic complaint. Somebody might come in and tell you he is anxious and this is what he wants to be helped with. Then, you say, "What is it that makes you anxious?" You find out that this is a pattern of anxiety about relationships, let's say to women. So we might say that this might be the area responsible for the anxiety. Can we do something to understand your relationship with women rather than simply to decrease your anxiety by giving you an aspirin to take care of your headache, which is going to be back again in four hours?

The second criterion was the ability to demonstrate a give-and-take relationship with another person in childhood. To us, this was crucial. What does it mean to have a give-and-take, meaningful, altruistic relationship? If a child has been able to interact with another person by being able to make a sacrifice for the other person, altruistically, that child cannot be a borderline character, cannot be a narcissistic character, and certainly cannot be psychotic, because this aspect of having developed at the age of six, seven, or eight the tendency to be able to make a sacrifice for another person means sophistication, psychologically speaking, which is much more on the healthier side. The narcissistic character is not likely to be so open as a child and making this kind of contribution. We ask for instance, "Have you had a specific important relationship with somebody in your childhood?" Sometimes, patients say yes. "Could you give me an example?" This saying yes is not sufficient; we want a specific example.

Let me describe, for instance, a young woman of whom I asked that question. I said, "Do you have a friend?" She said, "Yes." I said, "Could you tell me something about your friend?" She told me about how they used to play together and have a good time and so forth. I asked, "Did you make a sacrifice for your friend?" She thought and thought about it, and she said, "Yes. When I was seven years old, my mother came and told me that my friend was sick and in the hospital. I was very sad about that and I wanted to go and visit her. My mother said they don't let children visit and you can't go because your friend is very sick. This lasted for about three weeks. Then my mother told me she had good news and I could visit Ellen now because she was very much better and they would allow children to go in. I felt so happy that I went up to my room, put down all my dolls on my bed, and then picked up my most favorite doll, which was a Raggedy Ann doll. I started to cry. And I said I have to give you up because you are my favorite doll, but you are going to be of so much use to my friend."

Now, a child who is able to make, at the age of seven, a sacrifice of such an important thing as a doll couldn't possibly, in my opinion, ever be able to have enormously complicated problems later on in life. Whatever the problems that she might have later on in life would be much more circumscribed, more specific, than the more global type of issues we have been talking about here, which affect the whole self or the character structure of the cases presented.

Now, to make doubly certain, we wanted to check with these particular patients and see whether the third criterion was confirming the evidence of the second one. If this client has been able to have meaningful relationships as a child, how does she learn to interact with us, whom she is meeting for the first time? The ability to interact in a flexible way with the evaluator, not necessarily submissively or compliantly but to interact in a give-and-take way demonstrates, I think, that this particular person has that capacity.

Now, we need two more things: first, a psychological

kind of awareness that the problems are psychological rather than a desire for a pill to cure the depression or anxiety or what have you; and second, motivation for change. For change, not for symptom relief. If I come around and say to you, "Cure my depression, you are the magician or therapist," that is not motivation for change.

Motivation for change is, "I know there are some things in my life that have produced this particular problem, but I can't figure them out and I want you, my therapist, to help me out." This is idealized language, I know, but the message is, "I have the pieces of the jigsaw puzzle that I have been trying to put together, but I can't. You have the know-how of how to put pieces of the jigsaw puzzle together. Let's work together. I'm going to give you the pieces and you show me how to put them together. Then, the picture might start emerging."

Dr. Masterson emphasized repeatedly, yesterday, the crucial importance of a working alliance which becomes a therapeutic alliance as we move along in the therapy.

There are two more aspects that are important. First is our own ability to formulate now, in our own head as an evaluator, a dynamic formulation—that the problem here is an unresolved oedipal problem, or an unresolved grief reaction or response to a loss and separation issue, or whatever, and to communicate that to the patient.

You might say, "You've come in because of anxiety. In my opinion, the anxiety is due to your earlier relationships with your mother, which are now interfering in your relationships with women in general. This is what makes you anxious and brings you here. Are you willing to work with your therapist in this particular area?"

Second, we want the patient's agreement to that. If the patient says, "No, thank you, give me a pill or something," I would say, "Fine, go to another clinic to get your pill." But if the patient agrees, and she usually does, then we have the criteria for selection. We have the specific focus on which to work on and which has been agreed upon.

One more thing about motivation: Because motivation is so important, we have developed sub-criteria for it. First, the ability of patients to interact with the evaluator. Second, the ability to give a truthful account of themselves. Third, the ability to know that their problems are psychological in nature. Fourth, to be curious and willing to experiment and try to make something different. Fifth, the ability to have realistic expectations of the outcome. And sixth, making a tangible sacrifice.

Now, let me give you an example for the last two. One is a patient who did not pass the fifth criterion—having realistic expectations of the outcome. I asked this young man, "What would you expect as a result of your therapy if we were to treat you," and he said, "the Pulitzer Prize." I said, "Interesting, so we have a writer here." And he said, "I'm a potential writer. "As a result of my treatment, which is going to tap on this great talent that I have, I would be able to write and get the Pultizer Prize." These were unrealistic, grandiose expectations that did not pass.

As for tangible sacrifice, we have a sliding scale in the clinic and we ask about the client's finances to pay for the clinic. A young man who came in with terrible problems in his relationships with women was getting $100 a week at his job, which was not too bad in the late 60s.

"How much shall we tell the clinic to charge you?" He said, "As low fee as possible because I have a lot of things to pay." I said, "Well, how much?" He suggested $1.00. I said, "A dollar? You make $100 a week and you pay $15 a month to your parents. You tell me that you have terrible relationships with women, and that is worth only $1.00? Well, I'll tell the clinic $15.00." "Oh, no, that's too much because I have to pay for my car and I have three different suits and I have these magazines and I have my record player." Forget it.

We said that it was $15, take it or leave it. Otherwise,

WORKSHOP: PETER E. SIFNEOS, M.D.   *197*

go to another clinic. Thank goodness we had the freedom to do that since there is no point to being forced to see people you know will not benefit from your treatment approach.

Another one is the timing. Let's say we have a patient who is available for psychotherapy. We have a therapist available for you on Mondays at 9. No, that's after the weekend, that's difficult. Wednesdays at noon? That's my lunch hour. Friday afternoon at 4? That's TGIF. Anything on Sunday? No. Then, good-bye. If you don't want to make some kind of a tangible sacrifice to be there, then we are wasting our time.

So these subcriteria have been of great value. We have done a study on using these seven in order to accept or reject patients for short-term therapy, what we call STAPS, meaning Short-Term-Anxiety-Provoking Psychotherapy. To accept those patients, we need them to pass seven or six of those criteria. Seven is excellent, six is good, five is fair. Anything below that is unmotivated and we wouldn't accept them.

We picked up all patients, not only those for STAPS, but all patients in the clinic, and we asked the therapist to fill in this motivation about every third interview. We had some patients who were very sick individuals, but appeared to be unmotivated. They were given longer-term psychotherapy. This evaluation scale was valuable, too, in assessing the course of therapy. Let's say somebody had a motivation of one. After about six interviews, motivation becomes two. The therapist claims there is a change. After about 10 interviews, motivation becomes three. This is a prognostic sign of a successful psychotherapy. However, when a patient appears to have motivation of seven and then, by about the fourth interview, gets down to five and subsequently to two, beware.

There was an interesting example of this. We were doing what is called group control. One person presents a case interview to a group of us and we all discuss it. This was a young man who had a problem of anxiety because of difficulties in his relationships with men in authority. He had been offered jobs at two banks and he couldn't make up his mind which job to take. He became quite anxious about this.

The evaluators felt that this was only the tip of the iceberg, that the basic problem was his relationships with men and with a very authoritative father. He had a problem with the executives of both banks in terms of making a decision.

So we asked, "Would you like to work on this particular area? We don't know how much it would help your anxiety, but it might help your understanding." He agreed. In the third interview he said that one of the banks had withdrawn their offer, so he accepted the other one. And he felt better. At the fifth interview, he complained about the cold and the snow in Boston and expressed a wish to be in Florida, basking in the sun.

We told the therapist that motivation seemed to be dwindling here, but to keep on. It's unfortunate we don't have a way to inject motivation into people. Motivation dwindled and the patient stopped therapy. We lost him and it was one of our failures. As a matter of fact, we keep looking at our failures because they are often more instructive than our successes.

Question: Do people know in advance that this is short-term therapy?

Dr. Sifneos: No. What we would tell them is this: "As a result of your evaluations, we feel we could offer you treatment in the area that we have specified—namely, your response or sensitivity to loss and separation, which we know you have experienced in various situations. Are you willing to work on that?" The patient says, "Yes."

"Then we are going to help you do that over a short

period of time, once a week, 45 minutes." "What do you mean, short period of time?" "Well, I don't know how long it would take you to resolve these problems with your therapist. But it would be over a short period of time—namely, a few months. We don't do what James Mann does. He has 12 interviews with everybody. We leave it open-ended."

Some people have seven interviews; others have 10 to 15. If they appear to be motivated, but really are not, then longer-term psychotherapy might be needed with some of these people.

Our first study was the first controlled study on short-term dynamic psychotherapy. We selected patients, matched them according to age and sex, and designated the experimental patients. All were seen by two independent evaluators who set up criteria for outcome. The experimental patients would be treated right away, no waiting. With each of our therapists under supervision by one of us, we made doubly certain of the technique. Now the technique we can discuss later on if you like. The control patients, designated randomly because our secretary was matching them and assigning them without our direction, would have to wait until their experimental counterpart finished treatment in four, five, or six months. Of course, we wanted to see after that period what the control patients looked like. If Isaac Marks was correct, the controls without therapy and the experimentals with therapy would do equally well, according to criteria for outcome that I mentioned yesterday.

What actually happened was that occasionally we found that the controlled patient had symptomatic improvement. But none of the other criteria—interpersonal relationships, self-esteem, problem-solving, new learning development, new attitudes, work performance, ability to specify insight—had changed. However, symptomatic improvement did indeed take place. And if you look upon only symptoms rather than what lies behind them, under the iceberg really, then those who are so enthusiastic in treating symptoms with behavior modification or psychopharmacology, for example, do have their justification. I certainly am not saying they shouldn't.

However, I don't think the symptom is the important point. It is much more a more global kind of assessment of the patient's character structure. This is apparent, for instance, with interpersonal relationships. Thus, you might say, "My anxiety is much better but my problem with my father continues to be exactly the same." Or, "My problem that I have with my bosses continues to be the same, but I'm less anxious."

Of course, psychopharmacology—the use of antianxiety drugs—might have decreased the anxiety, but it would not have changed any of the basic aspects of the patient's character structure. So what we are saying is that we want more than a symptomatic improvement.

Question: But the target behavior for behavior therapy may be other than symptomatic relief. The target behavior may be better relationship with peers and better relationship with the boss.

Dr. Sifneos: If that happens, I would say, then, that behavior modification has altered not only the symptoms but also the basic character structure and therefore has been very successful.

Question: Has there been research comparing behavior with your approach?

Dr. Sifneos: No. And it has to be done. You would have to divide patients into four sections to receive short-term dynamic psychotherapy, behavior therapy, psychopharmacology, and no treatment respectively. Then you have to compare those four groups and see in terms of criteria for outcome which one has done best.

I cannot do this particular research myself because I'm biased and it's an ethical issue. If I see a person with certain problems and characteristics, I'm not going to give her psychopharmacological medication or behavior therapy when I know perfectly well what we have done with this type of person and the way our treatment has worked, and therefore I'm biased. On the other hand, you or anyone else might be perfectly willing to do comparison and, indeed, it is a study that has to be done—namely, comparison of various approaches with a homogeneous group of people in terms of what results we can obtain. Indeed, if somebody were to say I have used this particular technique that I define and in two interviews I have a better result in terms of the criteria for outcome than you have in your eight to 10 interviews, that's fine. I think we all will have contributed something.

Question: Would you give this type of therapy to children and older people?

Dr. Sifneos: As to young people from about eight to 15, the answer is that I don't know. I have been asking our friends in child psychiatry about this and they say that because the child's ego is in the process of development, you cannot grab hold and do this kind of alliance together.

The best we did was to start with adolescents at the age of 17. These were what I called emancipated adolescents— that is, young people who have solidified their ego structure. They were not the adolescents who are changing from day to day and are acting out.

As for older patients, we stopped at the age of 40 on our first study because we believed what Freud had said, that older people are too rigid, etc. He was wrong. We have found the over-40s a marvelous set of patients. There was a conference on aging in Washington at NIMH and I presented 18 of my patients between the ages of 50 and 84. Ten of those were people who had lost a spouse or

some very important person. The other eight had unresolved oedipal problems. I shall never forget one of them,
a delightful lady of 78 who came to us and said, "I want
some help because I want to get remarried. I've been
married three times and all my husbands were very nice
men and they all have died, but none of them measured
up to my daddy."

Now if I were planning to get married for the fourth
time, I would also want to find somebody almost as good
as my daddy. A 78-year-old lady talking like a 17-year-old
girl. It was a pleasure. She certainly met our criteria for
selection, with a considerable degree of flexibility. Obviously, it is ridiculous to talk only about young people.

But your question about younger people is of great
interest to me. I really don't know how to answer it in-
telligently since there is no literature and very few papers
that I know.

It would be of great interest if you could say that a child
from eight on starts having a consolidation of the character
structure, but that you're worried about how much the
anxiety might permeate the family setting and create some
problems. These are very interesting questions as to how
one would be able to deal with these youngsters, whether
one might have the mother or another member of the
family seeing somebody at the same time, and similar
questions.

I have spent a great deal of time on the evaluation, but
I would like to give one more example, which is somewhat
amusing.

I was an evaluator and a woman came in and told me
her roommate had been treated in our clinic. She said this
must be a wonderful clinic because her friend didn't have
to wait at all and now she was very happy after treatment.

Her problem was that she was anxious, depressed, and
procrastinating. She couldn't make up her mind whether
she should marry her boyfriend or not. This had occurred

in previous relationships, as well. She said, "I understand if I'm accepted there would be no waiting in your clinic." I said I didn't know whether she would be experimental or control since it was our secretary who made the assignment and some patients, unfortunately, had to wait for three to five months. She said, "I've been waiting for a long time so I hope I won't be one of them." She turned out to be a control and had to wait.

Six months later she came back. And I'm the evaluator to see what changes have taken place during the waiting period. So I asked, "How are you," and she said, "I'm fine." I said, "I remember you were quite anxious, depressed, procrastinating because you couldn't make up your mind about marrying your boyfriend or not, which was a problem you had in the past." She said, "Yes, but I'm not anxious anymore."

I said, "You know you're better. What else can we do for you?" She said, "Don't tell me I have to wait more for my therapy." I asked, "Why do you want therapy? Your symptoms are gone." She said, "Of course I want therapy. I'll tell you what I did. After I saw you last time, I went out and the secretary opened the book and said I would have to wait five, six, seven months. I was furious. I thought it was bias in this clinic. I have this long-standing problem. My roommate has been helped and I tell you I need help and then I have to wait for a long time. So I decided to take matters into my own hands.

"I bought a bottle of Scotch and went to my dorm. I got drunk and I said, 'Heads I marry him, tails I don't.' Heads came, I married him, it was the right decision, and I'm happy."

So I said, "Congratulations." And she asked, "When can I start my therapy? Don't tell me I'm going to wait for another six months." I said, "Why do you want therapy?" "Oh for heavens sake," she said, "of course I want therapy. I want to understand why I had the problem." Then, smiling, she said, "What if tails had come up, where would I be now?"

There was motivation, indeed. This lady was not satisfied with this symptomatic kind of change. She wanted a more basic understanding. There was the crucial point.

Question: Does the problem have to be formulated in psychodynamic terms?

Dr. Sifneos: No. We are psychoanalytically oriented department so our formulation is a psychodynamic one. I'm not saying that another formulation by a different kind of approach might not be applicable.

Question: It's just that one of the criteria you have mentioned is the ability of the interviewer or the therapist to formulate the problem in psychodynamic terms. If this were not possible, would the patient be rejected?

Dr. Sifneos: He or she would not be accepted for our research or for our clinic. But the patient would be referred. There are patients, also, who say they're not interested in our short-term psychodynamic psychotherapy and they certainly are free to seek help elsewhere.

Question: What about the use of videotape?

Dr. Sifneos: Videotaping is a way of reinforcing some of our observations for other people to look at and arrive at some conclusion. Our own research was done by a group of five of us. Two of us, acting more or less independently, would be evaluators. There would always be two evaluators who would see the patient, formulate criteria for outcome, formulate a dynamic focus, and then present their findings to the group so that all five of us could agree unanimously whether or not we would accept the patient.

Videotape is very helpful in this process. Let us say you have videotaped your own evaluation interview and that of an independent evaluator. If there is a difference of opinion between the two of you, all five of us can look at both of the videotapes and decide.

Question: As I listen to you describe your patients, I think there must be about 12 such people in the United States. Looking at those who are referred to me for therapy, I don't know when I last saw somebody like that.

Dr. Sifneos: You will recall that by altering our criteria for selection, we got 500 patients instead of 50 in the next four years. I think the reason is simple. We had given a message to the community that we were interested in anybody going to see a mental health professional, but he or she must be very sick. The message people got was, "For me, who have problems in my relationship with my girlfriend or father or whatever, to come around would waste your time. You should be seeing very sick people only, those people hearing voices. I'm not crazy. Therefore, I am going to talk with my friend about my problem." But the friend is not a professional. So the problem is perpetuated.

So in Cambridge it is chic for people to talk about their psychotherapy. A lot of them are students. And these students are perfectly well put together people, but in certain areas they have their problems.

Now people come to us because they know we are interested in their problems and we get all these referrals. So the people are there, but they have to know that we are interested. Or they may fear that if they come around and see any one of us, they would be there four or five times a week at $150 an hour.

Question: I would like to impose a different hypothesis. I was thinking about the criteria. A patient of mine, clearly a narcissistic personality disorder, came in one day and said he no longer had his coat. He said there was this man in the street who was poor and hungry and he took it off and gave it to him because he felt he, himself had been down and out and he wanted to contribute something to the world. And so he gave his coat away. He didn't make a big fuss about this, but it had been a pattern of his for a very long time. Another patient came in and said she only felt good when she was taking care of other people. She cannot do anything for herself. If she has anything, she has to give it away.

These cases are extremes, of course, and you can talk about flexibility of response and stuff like that. But I am wondering if there are people, perhaps in the upper-level range of the personality, who relate to the approach you are offering and bring in a problem of a very concrete nature that also has deeper issues. Like, "Should I marry my boyfriend or should I not," rather than the more diffuse kind of things we see with people who come in and say, "You know, I'm chronically depressed and my life is empty." I think an upper-level personality disorder might come in and say, "I'm having trouble completing my last year of school," or "I'm having trouble deciding whether to marry this person or not, and I have had trouble in my last three relationships." This does happen, so it's not just the 12 neurotics.

Dr. Sifneos: I agree. I might add that there is an enormous proliferation of health services at universities who deal with an enormous number of problems. Students have problems about this particular course or that relationship or something like that. That usually results in either a long-term psychotherapy recommendation or, "You know, my son had that same type of problem. Go back and forget it." Or I might hand out a pill.

Question: Have you had the experience of an individual whom you have evaluated going home and falling apart because of the anxiety that has been evoked?

Dr. Sifneos: This hasn't happened. We have had seven failures in the three most recent research studies that we did. The question refers to failures in terms of the evaluation. We spend so much time on evaluation that we make doubly certain that the patient is not going to fall apart as a result of any anxiety increase. If the patient does fall apart, we would have really made serious mistakes in our evaluation.

Out of those seven patients whom we have considered as being failures in our series, five resulted from our faulty assessment of motivation for change. One example was a patient we felt was highly motivated. However, one of the social workers who had seen the patient at intake said that at the end of the evaluation interview the patient was procrastinating: He stood in the doorway, not wanting to leave. She felt there was something peculiar here because the patient had done so well otherwise. Why this clinging quality?

We discussed and discussed it and concluded it wasn't really serious. That was a mistake; the social worker was right. This issue of a more dependent quality in the character structure emerged in the therapy and the therapy was getting nowhere. We considered it a failure since the patient was unchanged and had to be shifted into longer-term psychotherapy.

As I said previously, all the criteria are important, but motivation is, I think, the most important because it shows you the quality of the patient's ability to withstand that anxiety.

Question: Do you look for any particular characteristics of the therapists, themselves?

Dr. Sifneos: Yes, we have criteria for therapists, but as far as I'm concerned the most important one is that they have not been brainwashed into believing that everybody has to get long-term psychotherapy, like that psychoanalyst teacher of mine who said the human mind takes a long time to change. Well, some human minds may take a long time to change, but there are others that don't have to take that long.

At Harvard we have six departments of psychiatry at different units that are independent of each other, but they are all under the umbrella of the university. At my hospital we are particularly interested in psychotherapy and have a long tradition of psychodynamic psychotherapy and psychosomatic medicine because we are a general hospital.

We used to have a fellowship for people who had gotten their training in some of the other hospitals and then come to us for a fifth year. There was a young doctor who had gotten his training at McLean Hospital and done a lot of long-term psychotherapy of schizophrenics. He came to me and said he had heard about this short-term therapy and would like to treat a patient. We said, "Fine. We'll select a patient and assign him or her to you, but we will specify the focus. This is because of all the research we have done. You have to stay within the focus, read what the techniques are, follow the evaluation we have done. The members of the team will supervise you, hour per hour." He said, "Would you mind if one of my other supervisors supervises me since he also is interested in learning how to do supervision of short-term therapy." I made the fatal mistake of saying yes.

Two months, three months went by, four months. "How is Mr. G?" "He's doing fine, what a nice patient." Six months, seven months. "How is Mr. G? Why is it taking so long?" "He's such a nice patient." "But why is he taking so long? Usually, it would have been completed in five or six months." "Well, we are working. We are working hard and he is doing very well." "What are you working on?" "On his grandfather's death." And I said, "That is not the focus. We told you what the focus is. You're doing long-term psychotherapy."

Twelve months passed, the longest case we had on record. Finally, it was finished. I was one of the evaluators seeing the patient and he did very well on all the questions we have for outcome. One of the questions is, "How did you like your therapist?" He replied, "I liked my therapist very much, he was such a nice man. I have one question to ask you. Why was he so much interested in my grandfather's death?"

From then on, we said we were not going to have anybody else do therapy on our patients except us. In the last study, there were two of us, George Fishman and myself, who supervised all the therapists to make doubly certain that they were doing what they were saying they were doing. You see this is one of the problems of the anecdotal approach when you hear that such and such was done and then you find out that it wasn't. That's where the videotape is important.

Question: This question is about Dr. James Mann's work, which I found of special interest because it flowed out of my knowledge of Mahler and separation/individuation. What are your thoughts about his very structured 12-session model? I think it is very psychodynamic, yet it does not use primarily an oedipal focus, but rather a separation/individuation model.

Dr. Sifneos: Yes, that's absolutely true. Jim Mann and I have been together in many workshops. I have commented many times that he has not specified criteria for selection very clearly. He has approached it by establishing this very rigid 12-interview model. He makes it clear that scheduled dates will be met. Every time he starts a session, he says this is the 9th session, we have 3 more, or this is the 6th session, we have 6 more. This is the last session period. And that's the end.

So the structure is very defined. The criteria for selection are somewhat looser. And there is no systematic research on the outcome. But this ability to focus on the separation/

individuation and termination issue can be quite helpful.

The oedipus complex has been the focus of the last two research studies that we have done. The reason we have done this is because some people say that the therapy we do is only for people with unresolved oedipal problems. This is not true. A recent patient, for example, is a young woman in whom the evaluation interview clearly identified a loss and separation issue around the death of her father when she was 12. That's what we work on in the therapy.

The reason we picked up the oedipal issue was to have as homogeneous a population as possible. So I think some of these patients who have loss and separation issues are perfectly suited for this therapy. Yes?

Question: Are there sex differences in your group and would your criteria for males be the same as for females?

Dr. Sifneos: We do have more women in our series than we have men, the reason possibly being that some of the younger men might go to the Veteran's Administration and various other facilities. Still I think we would insist on a male patient giving us tangible evidence of a meaningful relationship with another person. If I cannot get a good enough example, I would consider a second evaluation interview as being in order.

Let me give you an example of that second criterion. There was a patient who came in who passed the criteria very nicely except that we couldn't figure out the second one—namely, one meaningful relationship with another person in early childhood. He had lost both of his parents and was brought up by his rich grandmother in Maine in a very isolated place. He described his grandmother as an ogress and gave us pretty good examples of how she punished him by sending him to bed without dinner and without dessert and all that kind of thing. She decided not to send him to school, but to teach him, herself, up to the age of nine. So he lived in this palatial home in this isolated setting with this terrible grandmother. And yet he related very well to the various people who evaluated him. Where did he learn that? Is this criterion possibly not as important as we thought?

So we felt we needed a second interview. Halfway through the second interview, I was getting the same story and I was really seriously thinking that maybe there was something wrong with that second interview. And then, in passing, when he was telling me again about his being sent by his grandmother up to his room without dinner, he said, "But, you know, sometimes her cook would sneak in and bring up a tray. She was an Irish lady and she sang beautiful lullabies to me." There was his mother. I said, "Why didn't you mention that to us? We're very much interested in this lady." He burst into tears. She had died when he was 10 years old. Here, indeed, was a meaningful relationship and we were absolutely satisfied that he met that particular criterion.

Now, let us go on to technique. The therapist is ready, the criteria have been established, the focus has been agreed upon, we are ready to start. In the evaluation interview, you have seen the beginning of a working alliance. Not always, but it is there when you get the patient to agree with you that he will work on this particular focus. However, working alliance and therapeutic alliance are a matter of degree. Therapeutic alliance, of course, is a much more intensified type of information sharing where the patient has all the pieces of the jigsaw puzzle, all the memories, episodes, etc. And you are the know-how specialist. Together, we are going to do this.

One difference in technique from what most of you might be doing in long-term psychotherapy is our picking up the transference early. Sometimes it comes in as early as the first interview. As soon as the patient has something

to say about you, the therapist, you must pick that up. I
find this is one of the most difficult things for trainees to
learn how to do. They avoid it.

You know the old saying: Wait until the transference
appears as a resistance. You can do this in analysis because you have all the time in the world. It appears as
a resistance in about nine months time. Here we don't
have time to do this. As soon as the patient says anything
about you, you say, "Now tell me what you're thinking
about."

There was a patient whose first session was rather
stormy. In the second session, she said, "It was kind of
difficult last time. Maybe you do more of the talking today
that I do. By the way, I notice that you have a new tie."
"What are your thoughts about my tie?" "I just noticed it,
don't make a big fuss out of it." "No, I'm interested in
your thoughts about my tie." "Oh, for heaven's sake, I'm
interested in talking." And then she said, "By the way,
I remember that my older brother used to have a tie."
There is the bridge between past and present, and it's
crucial. "What about your older brother?" "I had troubles
with my father and mother, but he always took my side
and he always talked for me." So you have the bridge—
the tie and the talking about an important experience
with somebody in the past who was viewed as a positive
person.

Then the patient referred to the fact that I had written
a book and was well known. "So who does that remind
you of?" "It reminds me of my father."

But we had the fundamental aspect of the transference,
and the transference is the tool. The ability to establish
the transference as a working tool is vital.

Another point to remember is the activity of the therapist, which is crucial. Too often, inexperienced trainees
don't want to say very much because of fear of giving the
wrong interpretation.

Question: What do you do in short-term therapy when you have doubts about the direction to take?

Dr. Sifneos: Short-term psychotherapy is more difficult because there are six or seven balls up in the air and you don't always know which one to pick up because they all appear to be important. It seems to me that one can have several options. If the therapist were to take a particular approach, then such and such might come while another approach might lead in a different direction. A patient may have a very interesting association when he has been talking about the transference. What do you do then? Do you get more information about this interesting association? Or is that association a way to get you away from the transference that you were talking about? It's a matter of judgment at the time which one to pick up.

You have to decide these kinds of issues and sometimes you pick up the wrong thing. That is where the videotape is helpful. Sometimes I have seen my tapes and I kick myself. Why on earth did I do this? But then you have an opportunity to see that this was a one-way street and got nowhere. Retreat and pick up the other side.

Question: Because of the selection criteria, I would imagine it would make it more possible within the psychotherapy to focus on a particular area. As a result, the areas of doubt would not be as numerous as in longer-term therapy, where there is no set goal in mind or set focus.

Dr. Sifneos: Yes, absolutely true. That's a very good point. Also, because many things happen, by the fourth interview we can be almost in the midst of what you might see after two years of ordinary analysis. The patients move very fast and very quickly. And with the transference being enhanced, things develop rapidly.

In order to make an interpretation, you have to have the exact words of what the patient has said. This reinforces the impact of the interpretation when you are able to say that you are repeating exactly what the patient told you. And sometimes it's useful and effective to show the videotape so the patient can hear it for herself.

Let me give you a very interesting example of a male obsessive personality patient, it's the first one that we moved into that area, which is somewhat more complicated, and we were not sure that this would be such a good candidate.

He was the apple of his father's eye and I heard a lot about this. However, his father was, one could say, jealous of his son's getting a Ph.D. The father had always wanted to get a Ph.D, but he hadn't, so in a sense he's competing with his father. Then I said that we hadn't heard much about his mother. He told me how his mother and father had had some problems and his mother, when he was 13 years old, would come around and confide in him. One day his mother woke him up in the middle of the night and told him that his father had become impotent. Then she said, "If you were only 30 years older, you'd make so much better a husband for me than he does." And he said to me, "I wanted to jump out of the window, not to commit suicide but to get away from this. But I also felt very excited about this."

I had asked him earlier what his mother looked like and he had described to me that she had dark hair, was very fresh, as it were, and was very beautiful.

About the seventh interview, just before Christmas vacation, he reported that he was engaged to be married and his fiancée was in New York. He was going to spend Christmas vacation with his fiancée and said that for just one week before the vacation he had his last fling. I asked, "What does that mean?" He said, "I had my last fling. It was just one affair for one week only. It was just the last fling and it was very exciting." It was with another student and I asked, "What did this student look like?" He said, "Oh, I know what you mean. No, she didn't look at all like my mother."

Now he had described his mother but he had also used the word that she was very *coquettish*. Not as common a word as one would expect. He said, "No, she doesn't look at all like my mother because she's thin and she has blond hair, not dark hair, and she's very coquettish." I didn't say anything. There was that unusual word.

I asked, "What was this affair? Was it a sexual relationship?" "Yes, but of course in the beginning I was impotent, then it improved, and then at the end it was fine." I said, "Of course, I would have predicted that." He said, "What do you mean?" I said, "Having sexual intercourse with a coquettish mother, of course, like your father had with her." And he, an obsessive patient, exclaimed, "Wow!"

Some people say that you take notes, you somehow establish a barrier between yourself and the patient. This is not necessarily true, but sometimes such a barrier can be evident.

A second-year resident, a very gifted young man, was videotaping a patient whom I was supervising. In the first session, they worked on unresolved oedipal problems. In the second interview, he said this patient was telling him that he was raking her over the coals like her mother used to do. "Are we going to have a mother transference?" he asked me. I said, "No, you're not going to have any mother transference. She's maybe using this to avoid feelings for you as a male similar to those she had for her father."

The sixth interview came around and he reported, "I have nothing to tell you today because she cancelled." I asked why. "She called up and said she had just awakened from a dream and it was the end of the scheduled hour, so she couldn't come." I asked, "What did you say? How did you deal with that?" He said, "I told her not to have dreams like that and to cancel the hour." I said, "That's not the way to deal with it. Find out what was this dream that interfered with her therapy."

After the seventh interview, he reported that in the dream she was on a beach, making love to this man from six in the morning to six at night. Actually, 6 P.M. was the end of her appointment. This man was wearing a white coat and had a red beard. The therapist also used to wear a white coat and he also had a red beard. When she woke up, it was 6 P.M. and she had misssed her appointment. I said, "Obviously, you dealt with the transference, didn't you?" He said, "Yes." I said, "Show me on the tape how you dealt with it."

What did I see in the tape? There was this patient sitting at the edge of her chair and telling him this erotic dream with an enormous amount of enthusiasm. And there he was taking notes. Obviously, what he was doing in the face of this strong countertransference was taking notes in order to protect himself. Then, I hear him whisper, "Well, we know your feelings for me, like your mother."

And the patient, who had been smiling, was deflated like a balloon. I say, "My God, is this what you call a transference interpretation? She is describing you and being with you in this erotic scene on the beach for 12 hours and you talk about her mother. In the second interview, it was her mother who was raking her over the coals." As you can see, this is difficult for trainees. The patient shows the transference and you take notes in order to protect yourself. But it is very important to take notes. I recommend it very highly.

Another value of note taking is to help you remember the exact sequence of the material during those 45 minutes, especially since there is so much happening so fast. Reviewing this material prepares you for the next session.

In addition, even if you are videotaping, you don't have the time to spend 45 minutes looking at each tape. If you want to write up a case, it's very helpful to have your notes to pull all the sessions together.

We have discussed transference, anxiety-provoking confrontations, clarifications, and, most important, past/present links, which is the use of the transference to bring up something that has existed in the past. For example, the good brother who was talking and wearing a tie like the therapist did now was brought into the therapeutic situation alive, between the two of us. Therefore, the patient can experience the feelings that existed in the past and continue into the present.

We have correlated the original criteria and motivation with how many times during the first five interviews of the brief dynamic psychotherapy the therapist was able to make a past/present link interpretation. If it has been done quite often during those first five interviews, it is safe to predict successful outcome.

Thus, if motivation is kept high, as we have done with our kind of subcriteria in keeping it high, and if you are able to make enough past/present link interpretations in the early part of the therapy, you can virtually predict that you are going to have a successful outcome in this patient.

Question: What are the criteria that qualify therapists to do short-term dynamic psychotherapy?

Dr. Sifneos: I have talked before about such criteria, but mentioned only the ability to know and not to be brainwashed. Yes, there are other criteria. One is that the therapist should know psychodynamic theory. If you don't believe there is such a thing as dynamic theory, then obviously it's very difficult to do this kind of work. That's why it would be interesting to see if someone with a different orientation might work in a different way and achieve successes.

So psychodynamic theory is one. Another is not being brainwashed in terms of thinking that everybody has to be seen in long-term psychotherapy. The third is having the curiosity to do something which is different. That is an aspect of motivation, of course. The fourth one is having the actual motivation to learn how to do this therapy. This was not true of the fifth-year resident I have mentioned who was going to do exactly what he had learned to do and had been told never to touch the transference. In this therapy, you have to learn how to touch the transference. That is a difference in technique.

And finally, a crucial aspect is supervision on a one-to-one basis and, if possible, on videotape.

I don't feel that therapists have to go through short-term therapy themselves and I don't feel they have to get an anaylsis just to become a good therapist. I know there are many people who have the ability within themselves to do this therapy as long as they are willing to be supervised and also have these prerequisites I have mentioned.

Formerly, we used to use these fifth-year and fourth-year residents because we felt they were more sophisticated. As a result of this example I have described, we changed out policy so as to utilize the younger ones who are much more open to do this kind of therapy.

Question: Do you evaluate the patient's capacity to perceive the therapist as good and bad? His capacity for whole object relations?

Dr. Sifneos: If people can tolerate good and bad interactions in themselves and in their therapist, I would say by all means. And that that is the emphasis of really trying to assess very carefully in the beginning. I mean people say if you see four people to evaluate you my God I mean what, you're already doing therapy. And it might be a shortcoming to have such an emphasis on so many people for research purposes.

Another criterion is the ability to express a certain amount of negative feeling. I remember once I was 20 minutes late for my interview with one patient because of an emergency. I came in and said, "I'm terribly sorry to be late." He said, "I understand that you doctors can have emergencies. But I also have some problems. You see, I am a very careful person and I came in half an hour early so I wouldn't be late in my appointment with you. Therefore, I would appreciate it if this effort were made by you, too." I thought he was absolutely right. He was telling me, "This is where I stand. I'm not going to be kicked around."

At times, the anxiety we produce results in a lot of feeling and anger, but the anger is not vicious hate. Rather, it is ego syntonic.

Question: How does one judge that the therapy is ready to terminate?

Dr. Sifneos: Interestingly enough, 50% of the patients are the ones who bring up the issue, saying something like, "Now I am handling things in a very different way than I used to. Where do we go from here?" If one is a long-term therapist, one might raise many other questions about unresolved problems. But we all have pregenital issues, or oral tendencies, or this and that, but it doesn't necessarily mean that these problems are so overwhelming as in some of the patients we see. So we let sleeping dogs lie, in a sense. We have done the work we set out to do. Let's see what happens now.

As for the other 50% of the patients, the therapist might say, for example, "You gave me an excellent example of how things have changed in reference to your mother. When do you think we should end?" I had one patient who was very amusing when I said that to him. He had given me a beautiful example of change and I said, "Well, when do you want to stop? And he said, "Stop what?" I said, "Stop what we are doing, short-term therapy." "Oh, no," he said, "I like it. And I have all these problems with this and that and that," and he goes into 20 minutes of a kind of blue funk. Then he started to laugh and said, "You know, I'm just trying to continue because I like it so much. But, indeed, what you are saying is true."

With those patients with the unresolved oedipal problem, therapy goes merrily along and often, with about 10 minutes to go, they say "Of course, this is our last session. I did most of the hard work. I needed you to coax me around and help in this and that and the other, but now I'm ready to go." With patients who have loss and separation issues, we have at least two or three more sessions to deal with what it means to stop after having done good work on this issue of loss. It's a little longer, but not a prolonged kind of issue.

Now we come to the question of outcome. We have mentioned the criteria for outcome that evaluators follow. We want the evaluators to give us specific examples of improvements. Let's say I used to have difficulty in my relationship with my mother and now my relationship is much better. "Fine," the evaluator will say, "give me an example of how it is better."

We use two independent evaluators in the beginning. Then, a new evaluator from the outside comes at the end of the therapy who knows nothing about the patient, along with one of the original evaluators. We rotate evaluators as much as possible so that we can have an entirely unbiased judgment. We try to find people who are as objective as possible, with no particular interest in demonstrating that this therapy is working.

Then the therapist goes down the list of eight criteria, one after the other. In terms of rating, if the patient gets a score of 11 to 14, he is considered as recovered, meaning that the problem doesn't exist any longer. A score of 7 to 11 indicates the patient is very much better, while 3 to 7 means a little better. Anything below that means that the problem is unchanged.

Using the criteria, one evaluator rates the patient, then the other evaluator, and finally we combine the two. Now that's only half of the evaluation. The other half is what we call SIP, Specific Internal Predispostion: What were the ingredients in this particular patient's vulnerability and in what way has this vulnerability changed by means of new defense mechanisms? How does the patient tell you that he used to have this problem and in what way has the problem now disappeared or become much better? You may recall my saying that in the beginning we paid no attention when the patient said he had "learned"—we thought this was just cognitive stuff, but thank goodness we put it down in that paper. We attributed this to their being students and talking about learning. Fortunately, we learned better.

The most interesting finding is the point about whether one feels happy about the changes (*joie de vivre*). They put it this way: "In this therapy I learned a great deal about myself. Now I can utilize what I have learned if I face new emotional problems in my daily life. Therefore, I have this power within myself, rather than having to look around to find Dr. Sifneos who treated me three years ago.

"We face emotional problems in our lives all the time. The ability, however, to utilize what I had learned in therapy now lies in my own hands. I don't need him or anybody else. That is really what makes my life worthwhile. I have it now, I have that capability myself."

How they do that is fascinating. They do it in the sense of, "If I am faced with a new problem, I start raising the questions that my therapist used to ask me. Now I ask them myself and I answer them." I call that internalized dialogue. "I am doing this within my own head. My therapist is here, I don't know if it's the right brain or the left brain."

I have an amusing example of one of my patients who came in for a five-year follow-up. She was one of the rare ones with whom we have had such a long follow-up. She came in and said, "I had this problem, Dr. Sifneos, and I was thinking the kinds of questions you would be asking me if I were seeing you in therapy." Then she shook her head and said, "It didn't work. But then I imitated your accent and it worked so much better."

I felt very very happy about that because it says that the therapist is carried in one's head as a problem-solver without the individual needing to find that same therapist or a new therapist. The quality of life now is much better because the former patient has things in his or her own hands.

11

Workshop

Marian Tolpin, M.D.

Dr. Tolpin: I understand we can do whatever we like here in the workshop. So I'm open to clinical material.

Question: I know how Dr. Masterson would proceed with a typical self-distorted case. He would divide it into borderline, narcissistic, or schizoid, and then there would be an approach based on that particular diagnosis and on whether he thought there was a chance for long-term work resolution of abandonment depression. What would your approach be if somebody comes into your office and you decide he or she has a self disorder?

Dr. Tolpin: I don't know that I want to talk about it so much as an alternative. It's not so much that the approach is an alternative. Some of the thinking is different. It is important to understand that Masterson has been thinking about this for a long time and has evolved his systematic approach to various kinds of psychotherapy: less intensive or more intensive, based on his classification.

Because self psychology evolved out of psychoanalytic thinking and was not at first applied so much to disorders

that weren't considered as indications for psychoanalysis,
the kind of very systematic approach that says you do this
in this event and you do that in that event is still evolving.
So I'm not going to be able to give you more than an
overview about how we go about thinking about something.

The first thing you have to do to decide whether there's
a self disorder is to make an assessment, which takes a
little time. Dr. Klein described a patient who had been
hospitalized and was ready to try out a rapid clinical assessment of what this person was like. But again, because
self psychology really evolved in connection with psychoanalysis, the thinking was about a long-term trial of
treatment.

But let's say somebody like this woman Dr. Klein described appears on the scene. You're a clinician and your
assessment is part psychiatric (phenomenological) and part
psychodynamic. You see the disorganization Dr. Klein
described. You have some idea of the long-term history
and the reason for the consultation, and you make a clinical
judgment that your patient is not schizophrenic, she
doesn't have a major depression, and she's not manic depressive, evidently. The clinician makes these broad judgments because most of us who have been trained in
psychiatry as well as in psychoanalysis have a foot in both
worlds—the world of symptom clusters and the world of
unconscious mental functioning, the world of manifest behavior and the world of what the behavior might mean.

The patient was in the hospital and somebody was going
to give her ECT, but many of us would agree that this
somewhat disheveled, disorganized woman might be functioning at a better level given an adequate degree of help
in the form of appropriate treatment. At that time the ECT
seemed to have no indication.

You make this kind of broad clinical assessment first,
even though this may not satisfy your wish or need for

exactitude. At first, you can make an evaluation of whether you are dealing with a self disorder (that's a very broad category) or with a more circumscribed form of self pathology.

Very often, people call you up and say: "I have an issue in connection with my job that I want to talk about with somebody." That's the manifest complaint. The person may come in and tell you a long history of job dissatisfaction. He may get into the whole history of something else, but nevertheless it's the circumscribed problem that brings him. So you have to make a clinical assessment of this. These are diagnostic interviews or diagnostic consultations.

It is the unfolding of that in the consultation, not so much with the old fashioned anamnesis, the old-fashioned case history. That's not umimportant, but you also get an overall clinical impression of what level this person is at, what level he has been at, how he responds to you, what his life consists of, and so forth. And you begin to form an impression. It's not in terms of borderline or narcissistic, but rather in terms of the state of the self.

However, we want to ask what kind of person this is to start out with. I think this question is very important because the kind of person this is can get lost in the pressures of trying to make a formulation. I know that our students at the Institute of Psychoanalysis in Chicago take the Child and Adolescent Psychotherapy that the Institute offers. It's an intensive course in psychotherapy over a five-year period. They have to do about 20 diagnostic assessments in the course of their training. And they have to make use of the metapsychological profile, or the diagnostic assessment scheme that Anna Freud and her co-workers worked out at the Hempstead Clinic. It is an incredibly detailed evaluation of ego functioning, congnitive issues, the psychodynamics, and the genetics. I could not do that in a two- or three-hour consultation. I have the freedom now not to have to do that. I would have to rely a lot now on my clinical hunches and impressions. It is not an exact science. These are clinical judgments that we make, which we modify, revise, and correct as we work with the patient.

Nevertheless, we have to fit people into more or less broad categories. The reason for this is that you have to know current diagnostic thinking if you're going to fill our forms, collect insurance, and live in the practical world. Then you can think more dynamically about the self. So, it's a struggle. You have to serve several masters. And I don't mean that in terms of just being practical. You have to have some notion, even if you question the classification system, that there are broad categories: For instance, the patient is either reasonably functional and belongs probably in a line where you have certain positive expectations or he may not be together enough so that you have to make a decision as to the kind of disorder for which a person belongs in the hospital (such as massive fragmentation, depression, panic).

For persons who come for analysis, you don't really make a dynamic diagnosis until you have enough information. You know they don't show up in the analyst's office as a rule unless they are reasonably successful individuals who are functioning very well. Briefly, Kohut's criterion was that you decide what's wrong with this person, you make a dynamic-genetic diagnosis on the basis of the evolving transference. Now that is not a practical way of making a decision if you are in a general practice of psychiatry, or if you are a psychologist or social worker doing therapy in a general practice and you do a consultation. You don't often have the luxury to say to the patient, "We will wait and see."

If you are an analyst and the patient wants analysis, you start four times a week, see what evolves, and tell the patient what you think in a reasonable amount of time. The implicit idea is that you have already ascertained that analysis or intensive psychotherapy might be indicated for this person. What you do if your practice is largely short-term or has a tremendous spectrum is different. You see your patients once or twice a week. You have a spectrum of people from those with serious thinking disorders (these belong in the psychotic realm—the self is severely impaired) to people with milder disorders.

You learn as much as you can about the basic theoretical orientation. If you're learning self psychology, you have to learn the basics and then practice applying them. And the basics, the clarity, and the explanatory and the therapeutic value, in my mind, all come out of a changed view of development—that normal development takes place in a matrix of self and other, and that there is never a time when there is not a (phase-appropriate) self.

This view of development is then translated into an understanding of childhood, adolescent and adult pathology. Psychoanalysis originally posited the notion that there is no object and no self, that there is no original experience of an "I" and a "You," a "Me" and "Another" even in a rudimentary way. This phase of earliest development was called primary narcissism: The baby, himself or herself, was without awareness of anybody else in the world.

This proposition is fundamentally changed in self-psychological theory. It so changed that it does not accord with any other theory on the present-day scene. That's one of the reasons for what I said about Dr. Klein's interview. With this hospitalized patient he did a test that, in essence, asks, "Can you be involved with me in a process?" It is as if Dr. Klein said, "You're in quicksand and here's my hand. Can you reach out and take it?" That was, in essence, the clinical test he did, and we would all probably do it in our own way. This is a brilliant and essential diagnostic feature of what you do (not how you do it in terms of the specific content of his interview). The general idea, that there is a test like this, tells you, relatively unbiased by a theory, that this person is capable of taking the hand of somebody who reaches out to him and possibly making use of it.

I emphasize that because the theories have all said, up until now, the inner person has never separated out of a diadic unit or progressed from the objectless stage posited originally by psychoanalytic theory. This concept is specifically part of the theory of Margaret Mahler, who influenced Dr. Masterson so much. It is part of virtually every psychoanalytic theory of development. It was the theory that existed from the beginning and all the schools of thought that developed from the original, including the dissenting schools, took the proposition of objectlessness as the basic assumption about fixations on early developmental positions. Hardly anybody knows this, but Mahler's theory comes straight out of Otto Rank. In a book that's not read much now called *Schools of Psychoanalytic Thought* (Holt, Rinehart & Winston, 1955), Ruth Munroe surveys up until the fifties every school of psychoanalytic thought, including the whole category that she calls the self psychology. So there's nothing new about the attempt to focus on the self. Munroe mentions Adler, Jung, Horney and Sullivan. In any case, Rank even used the terms separation and individuation.

The concept was that there was this unity and oneness. Therefore, the psychological task of development is to separate and differentiate. The clinician looks at it theoretically as what will foster, what makes it possible for that person to separate out of this fused unity, or this undifferentiated state. I think this is the core of Masterson's theory and of his technique. I should say in terms of this exchange, which I think is really valuable for both sides, that I learned a couple of years ago that it is almost impossible to really understand the workings of another school of thought unless one immerses oneself in it clinically, including in clinical supervision.

The reason for this is that theories are merely outlined

in books, but we learn through apprenticeship and supervision. So it's a clinical supervisor who says, in effect, "This is what the theory means. This is how you do it." And it may not even be any longer like the original theory. However, the field as a whole has been wedded to the theory that there is an objectless state from which the person has to seperate out. If I understand it, the whole issue about not fostering a rewarding-part object unit or an abandoning-part object unit is that the patient has to differientiate out of that into a real self that then can be an independent entity and be self-propelling.

Well all of this theory has been gotten around. No psychoanalytical theory is quite right, no theory is quite wrong. Each is a particular way of looking at things in a particular era. We decide about which theory, I think, on the basis of how attractive it is to us, personally. How much can we understand it? How useful is it clinically? Psychoanalysis is not a hard science so that you have to try to recognize what the choices are that go into the whole banquet that's around you from which to choose.

What Masterson and his co-workers have done is to get around the theory of dual unity. They don't take it very seriously, which is another thing that seasoned clinicians do. They work with the maps they've got; that's all that theory is—a map that says, "You're here." And, "This is more or less the route that you are trying to take." They know that the theory says that the diagnosis is objectlessness or that the person has not differentiated enough. And they know that they want to get to an independent, self-propelling, self-sustaining state. They work around the theory by taking it for granted that the patient connects: Here's this person outside, communicatively matching up with you, telling you that it's useful to think about yourself and not just about the wife whom you're trying to impress in a divorce settlement. And they haven't worried about the patient's presumed undifferentiated inner state and lack of separation between himself and the other person. Instead, in their interventions they have, in the view of self psychology, taken on many self-object functions that the person is lacking himself. That is the essence of the self psychological point of view. Because development, to get back to my original point, proceeds by virtue of an interconnectedness. That's not the same as fusion; that's not the same as a psychological nondifferentiated state. There is interconnectedness between the infant self and the others, the significant ones with self-object functions. These self-object functions, pure and simple, are all those things that we do in the course of bringing up children (the infant, the latency child, the adolescent, the young person), which children experience as a vital part of their own self organization. In more distant terms, self-object functions are all the parental activities that are vital for maintenance and restoration. Does that mean that the significant person out there is perceived only as a function, as the narcissistic extension of the self without any rights, needs, wishes, desires, feelings of its own?

In extreme pathology, yes. In some circumscribed pathology, yes. In normal development, no. While the adult functions for the child as an extension, for example, the child knows the parent whose hand he takes to reach the cookies is a real person out there. The two-year-old can't reach the cookie jar, so he takes you by the hand and lifts your hand up. You are the extension of him functionally so he can get the cookies because you lend yourself to his purposes. That is a self-object function that the child needs, wants. It may not be so vital for him to have the cookies, but he wants them and wants to be powerful enough to reach them. (I want to distinguish between needs and wishes.) That's an example of just one of the almost infinite number of times that the child expects you to function as an extension of him and what he needs and wants.

In his first version of self-object theory, Kohut, like others, said the child and mother are merged. (Everybody, including Kohut, uses theoretical terms from previous eras and assigns new meanings.) However, he realized that there is an independent self with its own initiative if others are more or less attuned to what baby needs to retain or restore psychological inner equilibrium. The baby is an "I," an agent, not a reflective "I," not a subjectively aware "I." I'm moving my hand, I'm crying, I have a call of distress, no. But the baby is an independent center with wired-in incapacities to relate to the outside world. What's the evidence for that? Daniel Stern in his book, *The Interpersonal World of the Infant* (Basic Books, 1985), sums up an enormous amount of research. In an earlier book, *The First Relationship: Infant and Mother* (Harvard University Press, 1977), he describes infant research that is extremely useful to read, which he calls the "dance," referring to the parent-child dialogue that is ongoing almost from the beginning of life. It would be "adultamorphizing" to look at the baby who immediately looks at the human face, follows the human voice, is attuned to the mother's smell more than to any other woman's smell, and then say the baby knows the mother or loves the mother. There was a theory of "primary love" (cf. Michael Balint). There is no love at birth, but connectedness is wired into the human being. There is a primary tendency to connect up with another human being. It is wired in from birth. The studies of René Spitz, back in the '40s, show that even though you can't say the baby knows the mother, the baby prefers the mother's face to almost everything else. The thing that the baby looks at most, with the greatest interest and the greatest energy-producing effect is the human face. The configuration of the human face is compelling right from birth.

It doesn't even have to be the human face as such. A mask with eyes, a nose, a mouth, or even the configuration of a forehead and two dots for the eyes will do. You move it and the baby gets lively and energetic. It's wired in, it's part of human equipment. It is only when this nucleus of an active, independent center is destroyed by massive neglect, as shown in the early work of Spitz and Bowlby, that you have a depressed, apathetic baby who might even die. There are, of course, theories about the baby's reactions and this takes us back to why self psychology is so different from other theories. Some theories say: "The baby is dying because of rage. The primary destructive impulses which are wired in have no outlet." Kleinian theory has the idea that there are mothering functions that modulate and buffer inherent destructive impulses of the baby. However, you could say from a Kleinian point of view that the baby is dying of its own self-destructive urges turned inwards.

The change in outlook for self psychology is that aggression, or assertion or whatever you want to call it (initiative, the cry, the thrashing around, the rage attacks) is certainly there if the person who is taking care of the baby doesn't come, doesn't respond, doesn't do it right. Self psychology says rage and aggression are part of human equipment and are used in the service of the self and its survival, its self preservation, if you will. Freud's early theory of ego instincts and self preservation tried to deal with this issue before he formulated an aggressive drive and the death instinct. However, this doesn't mean there is primary destructiveness. There isn't an oral cannibalistic stage of libido, for example, as far as we are concerned. Does that mean that we don't have cannibalistic fantasies or impulses? No, it doesn't mean that. The man whom Dr. Klein treated said, in effect, "If I can't get what I need to activate or actualize myself, I will submit to you by your raping me. You'll submit to me by my raping you. So I will binge on food, I will eat everything in sight cannibalistically in order to fill up in a displaced and substitutive way either

through what appears to be sex sadomasochism or moral-
ity. In other words, we are the human animal with all sorts
of capabilities—oral, anal, genital—which are not the
source of conflict or pathology in normal development.
The baby's healthy appetite is not the untamed unconscious of Freudian or Kleinian theory. Normal orality is
not part of a seething caldron of destructive urges that
have to be tamed.

All these theoretical points bear with immediacy on clinical theory. When you approach your patient, there is a
difference if you think they're a seething caldron of destructive urges that have not been tamed or if you think
that they have not differentiated out of the symbiotic union
with the mother than if your idea about them is that they
have not sufficiently established those functions needed to
maintain and restore the self as an independent center of
initiative with continuity in time and space, with purposes
and ambitions that are part of self-fulfillment.

It is different clinically to think those functions the child
needed at any stage were defective, distorted, erratic, in-
consistent. The case material presented by Dr. Klein was
a wonderful example of deficient parental functions. This
man had a very involved father and as a boy he was attuned
to the self-object functions of the father because the
mother was not there for him. The father was there for
the boy to placate, to absorb himself into, but the mother
wasn't there psychologically. Like any normal child with
good endowment, the boy turned to his father as an alternative. The father was enormously involved with the
boy. He was like a magnet, but the way he functioned for
the son was destructive.

Thus, you look at this person who comes into your office
as a person whose cohesive organization is basically impaired. This would be the classic vocation, I think, for
clinicians who are going to see a broad range of patients
who are not self-selective people and who walk into an

analyst's office. This man whom Dr. Klein saw, regardless of the fact that he was suffering, was a person in whom you're not so afraid that there was such an impairment to his self-cohesion that he was going to fall apart.

These are broad clinical judgments you are able to make probably fairly rapidly after your training and some experience. You wouldn't have thought of putting him into the hospital. That means this is a self-organization that, whatever its faults, or weaknesses, is going to hold together. On the other hand, you are able to recognize those whose self-organization is falling apart or failing. Some of that is perfectly overt and you don't need self psychological theory or any other theory for such an assessment. You know you can be an observing psychiatrist or psychotherapist who can see this person is hallucinating, or on a manic spree, or sitting in a apathetic torpor.

All the forms of diagnosing mental illness you've learned in your training are relevant to assessing a self-organization—determining whether it is not adequately cohesive or "together." Although some forms of "fragmentation" may turn out to be biological problems, it doesn't make any immediate difference what they turn out to be. You have to recognize that they are profound impairments of self-organization and you get them to one side and then decide on management. Now the whole other group is a continuum of the self that is sufficiently together.

You've got to make your diagnostic assessment, but you have to be open to the possibility that it's off. You can organize self pathology according to the extent of the weakness of cohesion. For example, at one end of the spectrum is the person who falls into a state of abject humiliation with the slightest setback and deflation, or who becomes totally depleted and depressed from a setback. That is a severe form of weakness, and there are cases all along the spectrum.

Question: Does the therapist have a personal interest in the patient?

Dr. Tolpin: Any therapist who's going to invest any time and effort into his or her patient has to have some kind of attitude and investment other than making a living. That makes it a meaningful personal encounter. That doesn't mean that you hold hands or you're a cheerleader, but you have an attitude, which is why people come to you. They come to you as an expert in an attitude towards human beings who need help.

That is what you want to convey in a first encounter by your attitude. It's not so much what you say as the way you say it. So everything that Dr. Klein did I would say was indicated. My only question was about how he did it.

Question: How would you formulate what Dr. Masterson calls the rewarding-part object unit?

Dr. Tolpin: Let me make sure I understand the concept. The rewarding-part object unit is that this person has gotten secondary gain out of being an individual who is nonfunctional. The way I would conceptualize this is: This person has been in a chronic situation for years in which her basic needs for recognition, firmness (firmness is a self object function), encouragement, limits, etc. have been ignored. As a consequence, the pattern of a chronically unsatisfying and unsatisfactory relationship with the parents has gone around and around in a vicious circle, with the consequence that there is not that inner core with enough glue for her to be an independent center, a cohesive self. Everybody would conceptualize this differently, but most people would say the intent of Dr. Klein's interventions, the reason that he made them, and their effect were sound.

In my view he acts as glue for the patient and there are different ways of acting as glue. He also starts up with parental self-object functions that she never had a chance to internalize because they weren't sufficiently there. I'm sure the parents said, "Get up and get yourself dressed and get yourself together," but the girl is so neglected, unrecognized, shunned, and without impact that nothing from the parents can really be taken in that acts as inner glue. It isn't because you're supposed to be a glue giver. It is because the patient makes you into that when you provide enough.

It's essential for you to know that I do not mean that you give self object functions. You are not "empathic" and thereby giving the patient something. You make clinical judgments that have some sound basis and those judgments are the self-object function. You make a judgment that: "Not only does the patient not need hospitalization and ECT, but that would be further undermining her sense of being able to take care of herself." Those are judgments that the patient experiences, conveyed by you in your person to them.

That's why these encounters are crucial. A consultation is a consultation depending upon who's doing it and what he or she understands and conveys to the patient. I'll give you a quick example of this. One of the first follow-up cases in the psychoanalytic literature was written by Helene Deutsch, published around 1954. She wrote about some adolescent or late adolescent/young adult patients who were resistant to treatment, complained all the time, told her she was full of it, and said her theories were ridiculous. And lo and behold, much to her surprise, some of these people have written to her in their adulthood and they have stabilized. They were people with serious character problems.

They had stabilized and were getting along well and they wanted to come back and talk to her. And one of these young women came back and Helene Deutsch said: "I can't understand it. You were always telling me how terrible the treatment was and how ridiculous everything I said to you was and complaining about the theories." The woman responded, in effect, "Your theories, Dr. Deutsch, were ridiculous, but you were something else."

Question: In your model, where does the autonomous sense of self develop?

Dr. Tolpin: That's a perfectly fair question. In fact, I say it's not a libidinal phase model, not oral, anal, phallic. It's not that you can differentiate out of oneness and have to suddenly confront your smallness. That's the Mahler model. Instead, each phase of development is the development of the self as a cohesive unit in time and space, with continuity and purposes and urges. The emphasis in self psychology is actually more biological in a sense than earlier theories in that it includes everything that's wired in. So the idea of an emerging "I" is wired in and we know when it occurs.

Question: We talked about that sense that sets itself, for example, when a 14-year-old comes in and says: "I am John Smith." He doesn't like school, he doesn't like this, he doesn't like this.

Dr. Tolpin: This is heavily dependent on wired-in cognitive development. We know about cognitive development, and we can tell you exactly when there is more of a sense of "I" than the neonate has. One of the experiments that's done by people who study self development cognitively is this: when the eight- or nine-month-olds, or children a little younger than that, look in the mirror, they love it. They get very animated and excited, but they seem to think that they see another being. There seems to be an alter ego or another person possibly out there. Around 15 months of age, if while the baby is asleep you put a mark on her forehead, you can see that when the baby looks in the mirror, instead of having all this animation and interest, she immediately touches her own forehead, which she sees reflected in the mirror.

Primates, chimpanzees, get just as excited as younger infants when they see themselves in the mirror. However, they never get to the body-self recognition experience of the 15-month-old, "This is me," as it were. That's wired in, you can see it. Unless there's an impairment in constitutional basic equipment, self-recognition emerges on schedule. This nucleus of wired-in, unfolding, emerging capacities is crucial for knowing, "I am I."

Question: Are you saying that the time when you mature in the cognitive apparatus has a great deal to do with it?

Dr. Tolpin: It has an enormous amount to do with it, and it has everything to do with it in this sense: If it isn't there, you cannot build it in. You cannot differentiate out a self unless there is a nucleus of these inbuilt emerging potentialities. Of course, these need to meet up with an "expectable" environment that fosters and facilitates emergent development of a self. Psychologically, you have to have parents who say, "This is Tommy," to give the effective and the "oomph" part to the "This is me" experience.

You don't just have an automaton that says, "This is me," because there are all these affective, surrounding, self-object experiences that are always intermeshed with cognitive development. Cognitive development can go on and emerge according to its time and place. And yet there can be something so impaired in the self-object unit that it's a flat, "This is me." Or it is a depressed me, or an empty me, or a lethargic me.

Question: One of the things Heinz Lichtenstein spoke about is the early identity being quite full as to the reflection of a mother's delight. How the mother perceives and receives is how that infant is going to see himself or herself throughout the life cycle. Treatment can lead to transformations, but that fundamental identity is going to be maintained throughout life.

Dr. Tolpin: You mean in terms of the reflection of the mirroring mother? Heinz Lichtenstein was very creative. I just cited him in a paper on female sexuality. He had one of the great insights into that issue, but it also has to do with selfness, so I'll mention it in this connection.

Freud thought everything was oedipal. Then he encountered a group called, "Women of Elemental Passionateness." That's not a compliment, although I used to think it was until I understood the context. Freud said there was a group of women who wanted soup for logic, logic and dumplings for reasoning. He found that treating was like writing on water. He thought they wanted the father's baby (soup and dumplings) and they didn't get better when he told them their symptoms, their rages, their masochism were the result of an unconscious wish for the father's baby, and not for the therapist's baby.

That's the theory you heard elaborated into Dr. Sifneos' short-term intervention. They didn't get better, so what did Freud do? This is the paradigm in psychoanalysis, he said: "Sometimes you say the patient's wrong." That, unfortunately, is a paradigm also, but this time he said the theory is wrong, so he changed the theory of the wish for the oedipal baby.

He said: "The trouble with these women is that they are enraged and they are narcissistically injured." This is the first idea about narcissistic injury. They want to be men. Women are enraged because they don't have a penis. Possessing a penis is the ultimate for them and they are enraged at their mothers for not giving them the penis. This is why they have such bad relationships with men and women and regard themselves as injured.

Then a whole era of psychoanalysis, another 15 years of psychoanalysis, followed. An era is approximately 15

years, which is long enough to try out new theory and see
its strengths and deficiencies. Again, a whole group of
patients didn't get better. Enter Melanie Klein. She said:
"I'm more Freudian than the other Freudians. The reason
these patients are not getting better is because the problem
in their development was earlier. It wasn't oedipal, it was
earlier, pre-oedipal."

Now just think what would have happened in psychoanalytic theory if somebody had come along and said: "It
wasn't earlier it was later." It had to do with these patients'
latency, or their adolescence or their young adulthood.
Just think what we all know now. What if somebody had
said in the early years of this century that the opportunities
for women are so narrow, what is expected of them is so
restricting and so distorting of normal development, that
it must be *later* that a little girl turns into a withered
woman? George Bernard Shaw says in one of his plays, in
one of his most acid comments: "Girls wither into women."
What if we had recognized that girls wither into women
because of the kind of distorting pressures that shaped
preadolescent and adolescent girls' psychological makeup?

And what if we realized today that earliest development
is not all-determining? People turn into drug addicts, or
into delinquents, or steal a kid's gym shoes and kill him
for them because of the atrophy of the personality structures when there is no chance for psychological growth
with the enormous limitations of opportunity for health-
promoting self-object functions in adolescence and young
adulthood.

Instead of recognizing the later blows to healthy development, we had the "It has to be sooner" fallacy. Like
almost all other analysts, Heinz Lichtenstein also assumed
earliest development was the main influence in pathology.
Now it is possible that a lot of people still emerge from
infancy with an intact nuclear self, and later deprivation is

the major issue or, at least, of great importance. The nuclear self needs sustenance.

The pole of the grandiose exhibitionist self says, "I'm great, look at me." And the pole of the idealizing self looks up to the idealized parent and says, "You're wonderful, you're big and you're strong, and because you're strong, I'm strong, too, because I'm like you or I'm going to be like you." With some response to these basic configurations, they can still come out with a reasonably intact self. How can we measure that? A lot of these kids go to headstart and they do great because the self is responded to. The minute they stop going to headstart and go back into their regular world, they can no longer do well. Their needs for mirroring for ideals, for alter ego experiences, are no longer responded to.

So the theory and your attitude about it are all-determining. If you look at a child who comes in and you think, "Well, it all happened in infancy. That's printed forever," you're going to have a much more limited range of possibilities in your mind for this primary experience of self-development and self-establishment. One of Lichtenstein's most interesting contributions came in the 1970s and helped demolish a myth in psychoanalysis. The myth was that sexuality and the capacity for orgasm are the Utopia of what is called "Genitality" and "Maturity." Lichtenstein and a few other writers said, "No, sexuality is enormously self-affirming. Sexuality gives you a sense of 'I am I,' and that's why it is so important and can serve that function. It doesn't have to be part of a line of development that says you're mature if you have sexuality and orgasm. That's not necessarily so. You might be self-affirming."

That didn't really get integrated until Kohut came along and said about sexuality that it can be used "defensively," or self-protectively, to buoy up the self and to improve cohesion.

The reason it became so important is that you can affirm yourself through sexuality. In response to my question, "Where did this hand turn," someone here said, "He turned to art, and art then became himself." You can turn to your own erogenous zones or to somebody else's erogenous zones when you are failing, when you are depleted, when you are depressed, when you are abandoned, neglected, or caught up in a system of "rewards." Rewards do not foster self-development. In Masterson's sense, rewards mean you're being rewarded for being a passive compliant child who goes along with parental neglect. Or you are being rewarded for being the self-object function for a sadistic father who has to be heightened by his child all the time to maintain his faltering cohesion.

When you're caught in something like that, you always have yourself and your erogenous zones to turn to. That is basically the meaning of the defensive use of sexuality, i.e., sexualization, in self psychology. It is one of the most powerful defenses, in the sense of defense meaning anything that protects the self and its cohesion even if it is further pathogenic. It has as its purpose the protection of a failing or faltering self. You turn to yourself or to somebody else and you get involved in all these oral, anal phallic perversions that are used in place of genuine self-sustaining functions that you can't elicit from your world.

While defenses serve to protect the self, many further undermine the self-organization. Defenses become addicting. Why do we get addicted? Because we manage to preserve some aspect of this wonderful self, this wonderful "I." Again, that's where the psychological part of the theory comes in; it would be just dry if you stuck only to the cognitive part of the "I."

Sometimes, one uses a word like "contain," which immediately suggests Bion and another whole set of theories of infantile development, all of which evolved in trying to deal with these clinical issues. The fact is that all of the theories are right in the sense that they touch on the missing inner functions that hold the self together. In Dr. Masterson's framework, they touch on the habituation to not activating the self, not using the capacities you have. You are always trying to say, in essence, the patient is caught up in this web of pathological object relations that doesn't allow him or her to use the capacities he/she has. Your approach to the patient, then, fundamentally is that you, the patient, are going to have to understand those defenses. I'm going to have to help you understand them by undermining them and confronting you with them so that you can use and activate yourself.

I have no objection to this approach, except that I would translate it into the idea that the borderline person who is caught up in this series of defenses has not yet really developed the structures needed to be self-activating. However, you see them as a potential. Some of the capacities are really there as long as there's "glue." What serves as the glue is not ingested. The glue is there in the consultations with the therapist and it's there in the ongoing treatment. Thus, both theories here basically deal with the same issue even though they're formulated very differently as I've gotten to understand more of what Masterson is talking about.

My particular emphasis, not incompatible with yours, is that you have to understand that you can't activate the self by telling people about their defenses until you also give them an opportunity to first hold onto their self-object functions and then facilitate their gradually taking enough in so that their self becomes more firmly organized. Do we have a real difference there?

Question: How does this view compare with Alice Miller's?

Dr. Tolpin: I have the same issue with this outlook that I would have with Alice Miller, who says you have to mourn that self that was in your terms caught up in the system of rewarding self. The patient is an extension of the parent that says, "You're great," and is great only as long as he/she is connected with the parent and the way the parent wants it.

This is what's called total immersion. She says you have to mourn that self, and self-object theory says you don't mourn anything unless you build up something within yourself which makes it possible then to lose it. You can't tell a person to mourn and give up a faulty attachment until there is a foundation and the person is not in quicksand anymore, psychologically speaking.

In my view, you mourn in treatment because you are capable of losing someone important because you have the self-object functions that enable you to mourn in therapy. You mourn because you are engaged in the self-object unit that was previously disruptive and never adequately internalized. Thus, the original psychoanalytic theory put the cart before the horse. The theory says you have to mourn in order to overcome the loss, whereas self-object theory says you have to firm up the self with the adequate functions in order to be able to stand to lose anything.

By and large, most people aren't interested in theory. They are clinicians and they want to know how to do it, which is quite legitimate. However, those who worry about theory realize there are fundamentals that organize your clinical approach.

Some of you have asked why we should spend time saying this analytic theory is wrong or mine is right. I hope we're not doing that, particularly since there is so much overlapping in outlook and intent with the Masterson view and the Kohut view. People trained in Masterson's work see the similarities in outlook. I would like to describe what I think is the essence of the self psychological point of view that is different and adds a dimension that the Masterson outlook doesn't have.

First, I have said that a self object is a set of functions

needed for the development, the establishment, the maintenance, and the restoration of the self as a cohesive unit in space and time with independent initiative. I think that is implicit or inherent in many of the interventions in the Masterson work, but I think this explicitly spells it out.

Second, by virtue of fitting into a world of people who are attuned enough to the developing child, the child is an independent entity from early on. However, that is only by virtue of the self, with what's wired in, and the self-object functions interdigitating. In other words, we weren't born to be isolated. Independence does not mean we are born to be self sufficient. An independent entity is wired in to be connected up, to be vitalized and energized by the responsiveness of another individual. We can observe that from early on.

The third crucial difference in outlook, which is an added dimension of Masterson's work, is Kohut's concept of transmitting internalization. In a nutshell, you take over and make part of yourself, so that they belong to you, the capacities and functions first performed for you that are needed to establish, maintain, and restore the self. These functions can be divided into a whole group of categories that basically have to do with establishing and reestablishing homeostasis so that you don't feel like a lost little child. Sifneos' example of this is the loosening of repression in his model; his patient again became a child, but a lost little child.

You don't feel that there's a space or a wall between you and the rest of the world. You feel real, you take your existence for granted, you are sure that tomorrow you're going to look the same way as you do today and that the people in your world are going to look the same, and so forth.

Some of the functions have to do with restoration or maintenance of self-esteem. You fall down, but you are encouraged to get up and you are also soothed so that the injury to your pride and self-esteem isn't so great. As a result, a little bit of this is eventually taken over and made part of your own self-esteem regulating system.

But the crucial issue is that by first experiencing the functions of somebody else that are felt as part of your own organization, little by little you are able to take them over as you grow and as cognitive and maturational capacities and the right time come along. You don't take over regulation of your self-esteem as a two-month-old. You begin to take over regulation of your self-esteem around the second year of life when what emerges cognitively is that the child is beginning to make judgments about the quality of his or her own performance. That's wired in. You don't just get it because somebody else judges you. It's a tendency to have some notion about your own performance. And somebody out there is saying, "That's good" or "That's not so good." And that becomes part of a whole regulating system.

To use Kohut's analogy, which is a very powerful one, when you drink cow's milk, that's having the self-object functions of people you depend on. However, you ingest it, metabolize it, and build it into human cell structure, into human protein. You do not make it into cow protein; we can use cow protein only by breaking it down and changing it into human protein. It's got the amino acids in it that we need to manufacture human protein and our body is able to do that. That's what transmitting internalization is.

You hold onto your parent's hand when you cross the street and you feel a sense of safety and security and organization and sureness that you're going to get to the other side. In one little function, like holding onto your parents and feeling that secure, guiding, affectionate parent's hand, a whole bunch of qualities are experienced that become organized from cow protein—the parent and what he or she is doing for you to your taking it over and making it into human protein in your own cell structure, transmuting internalization into capacities that you need for your own self-organization to feel capable and effective and able to cross the street. I'm using that just as an analogy.

I would say also that the reason Kohut's work is so different in terms of emphasizing transmuting internalization is that he came out of a tradition of American ego psychology that emphasized all sorts of esoteric things like structure building. It all had to do with internal mechanics like how you tame impulses and drives. Yet he transmuted this American ego psychology emphasis on object relations in taming drives into this basic idea of how you acquire the capacity to feel real, to be real, to pursue your own ambitions and goals. That's a whole area of self psychology that is really important to pursue.

I hope I have answered your question about what a self object is. Think of it as drinking cow's milk and turning it into your own protein.

Many therapists ask what the technique is like. I saw Kohut for supervision consultation on a number of cases, as did many other people who worked with him. Whenever I said anything about analytic technique, I always thought he was sort of curling his lip. And I finally figured it out. I think this is an unhappy chapter in psychoanalytic theory, that there isn't a technique. The method of treating a person is to try to understand as much as you can about what makes that person tick, how he's put together, and what's wrong with him. Then you translate your understanding into interventions of which there are a whole range.

Question: In other words, you're acting this way when you have the capacity to act in another way.

Dr. Tolpin: Exactly. There are a whole range of explanations. See I think confrontations is a bad term because many confrontations have different content because they come from different theoretical framework. It's a term that's misunderstood, but you know what it is and that's what's important. But there is a whole spectrum of interventions. For example, you can say, "You are experiencing me this way and I think you continue to experience me this way because of the following . . ." and you make a formulation which is an explanation that tells the patient about the origins, the genesis, and the pathogenesis.

Now that's what is meant by interpretation. But that's just one example on this spectrum of explanations. That's what "technique" is. Technique as it evolved in psychoanalytic writings ended up to be this caricature of a person who deals with human beings, as with caricature of the analyst in *Portnoy's Complaint* where the monkey, Portnoy's girlfriend, says she knows her analyst is alive because he has an answering machine and only somebody alive would have an answering machine.

Question: I have a new client whom I'm uneasy with because I don't know how to classify him and I don't know how to work with him. I keep on trying one thing or another, but I don't have the sense that I have any real understanding.

He's a 29-year-old white, upper-middle-class, Jewish, professional man, a lawyer. He came to me with his second major depression. He doesn't seem very depressed to me, perhaps because he's on an antidepressant. I asked him why he came to see me and essentially it was prophylactic. He had had a major depression and his family had a major depression, he said. His father whom he identified with had had major depression. He himself had had one terrible depression while he was in school, dropped out, and then became a lawyer instead of an actor, but he didn't like it.

He had recently broken up with a young woman. She actually broke up with him when he couldn't commit to her over time. He then decided he had to have her.

His history with women is that he's a piner, in his own

words. He pines over women. His early memories are of wanting a woman, a girl in school whom he couldn't have and whom he could pine over. Very romantic.

And now he's pining over this woman. "If only she would let me into her life once more." He's very tall. He sinks down in the chair. My sense is he came to me referred by a very assertive mother and he was putting himself literally in my hands. He was going to tell me his problem and then it was up to me to do something. I found that I kept on asking him for more information since I was very vague on what he wanted.

Dr. Tolpin: Let me stop you right there because he's a totally different kind of person from Dr. Klein's patient, but with a similar kind of what you call defense. The "I'm here, do something for me." So you stop right there. You know now some people need to be educated in this day and age. One of the outcomes of this conference is that you're going to realize that many lawyers don't want to be lawyers. They want to be artists or actors or something similar.

Question: But I thought that's not bad. You have a so-called major depression and you can't be an actor, but you go to law school and become a lawyer.

Dr. Tolpin: In other words, there's a lot to this person. He has a lot of stamina, get up and go. He has a depression, but he also has some bounce, some reserves, some flexibility.

It seems to me that the starting point is to formulate to yourself what this means in terms of the therapy and then tuck it away in the back of your mind. I think it's too soon to say anything to the patient because the rest of the diagnostic work is going to help you formulate what you want to say to him. But you see that he's just sitting there with the idea that this is another consultation, like about the drug. You know he was put on the drug because he has this symptom and he expected the doctor to respond. The doctor did and gave him medicine, right?

You know that that's not how it works here. So go ahead.

Question: I had confronted or at least approached him with, "It seems unclear as to what you want to do here." I asked him to clarify his goals and I wrote down what he said while he was there. I also said that I had the sense that he was presenting himself to me and that he wanted me to decide what to do with him. I wasn't sure what kind of a reaction I got from him. I couldn't quite read him. It sounded like he was agreeing with me, but he also looked a bit off put and the following sessions were different.

Dr. Tolpin: I think that's a good place to start because that's the issue you feel you didn't confront. The way we would look at it is as a diagnostic question; whether you're dealing with a borderline with infantile features or someone who is more clearly a narcissistic.

Question: He told me that he had been this very bright boy, but that he wasn't really top notch.

Dr. Tolpin: The man tells you about his great expectations of himself, that he hasn't lived up to. He says on the one hand I have all these great expectations and was supposed to be this and that, but on the other hand I feel like a fraud. This is classical description, incidentally, of where Kohut started out with some of the people who have so much, but they feel fraudulent.

The psychoanalytic literature, from Freud on, is filled with cases like this. The field has struggled to understand these cases. Freud said many of them were wracked by success, that they had unconscious guilt because they were successful. That's the theory that Dr. Sifneos is using. They had to undo their success. Some of them even have to get punished for their success—be in a bad relationship or be rejected or wreck their career or not pursue their career.

But that didn't work with a lot of patients. So there is a whole group who formulate this problem in terms of destructive introjects, etc.

Kohut came along and said that maybe this is the kind of person who has this terrific endowment, lots of skills and talents, lots of ability. You look at the health of the personality first. You have to work hard to do that if you've had psychoanalytic training. If you have psychoanalytic training, you first think that he is borderline or narcissistic. You don't think what Kohut thought later, that this is a great guy. There is really something to this person.

So you have an overall impression that there is something to this person, he's achieved a lot, he had ambitions he had to give up, he feels fraudulent, he's sort of slumped there in his chair, passively.

Question: He has a sense of humor, however. He reported an incident at his own expense. When he was flagellating himself mentally, he called up his friends and one of them said, "You know what you need, Mark, a bigger whip."

Dr. Tolpin: So he told you an enormous amount. It's not as though he didn't give you the information. He's not just passively slumped in the chair saying, "I'm depressed, do something for me." He told you a lot. Why? Maybe because he has the expectation that you are going to tell him something of use to him. That's the other side of this notion that he is presenting himself as such a passive person and not taking responsibility for himself. I think that you do a tentative formulation of all the things I am talking about, including what seems to be some of the health and strengths of his personality, and you tell him about that. Or you say, "I have the impression that you have a lot of drive and you have succeeded in a lot of things and that you have ability, but there is this distress you have in terms of thinking yourself great on the one hand and a fraud on the other." The problem is for you to put it together and for you to know what to tell him.

I would wonder, with a patient like this, if he needed to be asked something about his expectations of therapy. What did he know about therapy? Who referred him to you? Someone you had helped?

Question: The mother of someone who had heard me lecture on borderline disorders.

Dr. Tolpin: Somebody said, "Here is this terrific therapist who knows all about people like you. Go see her." Right? So he's already got a transference to you. He's telling you a whole inner story about himself that's really very meaningful. It just unfolds spontaneously. So you say to him, "What are your expectations of therapy? What do you know about therapy?"

This isn't a person who is going to continue to sit, I don't get the impression that this is a person who needs that kind of intervention. I don't know what he needs to get you to have the feeling that he's going to enter into a collaborative work with you, because he already had. You know he's already doing what a patient is supposed to do. He's telling you a lot about himself.

I'm not really quite clear at this point what it even was that made you feel he was so passive. He's telling you about himself. What more do you want initially?

Question: He's crumbling physically. It's more of a sense I have and when I said it he agreed with me . . . that sense of himself. But he doesn't act, he actualizes, he becomes a lawyer . . . but it was just that there's something I can't put my finger on that's going on.

Dr. Tolpin: He was put off by what you told him, but that didn't come out. This is why I said the initial consultation or the initial work is so important. Some of your interventions may lead to subtle responses, but I don't know that you're differentiating a borderline from a narcissistic person when you do this and the patient is put off. I think it may be the awkwardness of your intervention, that you're saying to a person who has come to you for help that he is not really taking responsibility for himself. He has come, and by coming he has taken responsibility for himself. Find out what he expects.

Question: I asked him. He said that he thought that he could get a new perspective about some of the things that were happening to him. Indeed, some of the things I said in the sessions had given him a new perspective.

Dr. Tolpin: Is that a test of a possibility of getting into a therapeutic alliance?

Question: Yes.

Dr. Tolpin: It is. I think for purposes of discussion I've made a sort of quick formulation, but that may be too facile and I would want to test it out. Tentatively, I would say that, I wouldn't be that worried about an accurate diagnosis here because he's not in that part of the continuum that's falling apart, he's not where you say, "I'm not even going to suggest psychotherapy for this man. He seems too tenuous, too badly put together, too in need of shoring up. Let's see what happens with some strengthening interventions right now." After all he came with a major depression and he's on medication. Let's not forget that.

He's already established himself in a part of the spectrum where you think you can do psychotherapy. And he has also established himself, in my view, as a person with a self-esteem regulation problem. He has not been able to integrate into a cohesive sense of himself the great self and the self that is so subject to failing and therefore has a sense of fraudulence about itself. He is not that great self, although that great self is part of him, but not modulated, not integrated. Nor is he the totally defective and fraudulent person. But that is also part of him.

So, tentatively, I would say to somebody who came to me for consultation about this patient that it sounds like a treatable problem, like a self-esteem disorder. However, you have a person who has a major, major area of depletion or collapse or weakness and he's on medication for depression. Let's try to understand what that's about. You have to really consider this. Is he okay right now because he is on the medication?

In good time you will know all about severe pathology or the phenominology that leads to the differentiation between narcissism and borderline, and so forth. But you can leave it aside for the moment and be open and let the patient tell you more about himself or herself. You don't need this kind of pinprick test to see if the patient feels. You'll find out about it, I think, if you are more open in your expectation.

Question: Dr. Tolpin, the reason I can empathize is because of my own conscious. What I like about Masterson's differentiating early on in the therapy relationship is that it's been very helpful for me to be able to at least globalize largely borderline and narcissistic into rather large gross consultation approaches. It doesn't mean that I'm rigidly in one camp or the other, but at least it gives me a sense of bearing.

Dr. Tolpin: I don't know that the intervention needs to be the pinprick method as I said. I think you can do the same thing that you've been trained to do, but with a little more awareness of what you expect from treatment, of your expectations.

Question: That can be a confrontation, in my opinion.

Dr. Tolpin: Fine. It's like saying, "Why are you here and what are your expectations?" It does have innumerable reverberations and it certainly reverberates with the basic issue that you want to find out about. Does the person just say, "You're the doctor, you tell me"?

Of course if somebody like that were in my office, I guess I would tell them something about what I thought and then use that as the test. But again, I think we're talking about basically the same thing and there is some subtle difference about how you do it. What is needed is to enter into a relationship where we explore what's wrong and what you, as the therapist, can do about it. With you as an active participant, if need be. If you feel that this person doesn't really know and you have to test out if he can be an active participant, then you tell him. You tell him what you think.

Question: On this case I think there's something interesting because you went through the intervention to figure out, I think this patient brings in a lot of things that I would want to ask more about. He was feeling something, he went to a doctor, he had medication for depression. What was going on with him? What did he expect? What did he get? He went into a relationship with a girlfriend, he lost it, felt something, and then had an obsession about her afterwards. Now he heard something about you and he comes to you. Obviously, he must have been feeling something, needing something, wanting something. I feel we want to know a lot more. My hunch is that the woman he's obsessing about is maybe just a front. The buddy relationship with you, if you understood him more and looked at him more, may be questionable. You may get a much better understanding as to why he is doing what he's doing and what he's really about.

Dr. Tolpin: It brings out how complicated this particular situation is. That's all the more reason you don't worry about that kind of confrontation right at the beginning. You have too many unanswered questions. You could even tell the patient that you want to explore the depression with him. You have to make some assessment of whether he came out of the depression because of the medication. That's a good assumption.

So this is one of those cases where it isn't because the patient has not been a very forthcoming individual. He immediately establishes that he's psychologically minded, that he's introspective, that he has some sense of humor, even though self depreciating, that he has a lot of assets and strengths.

You can make a treatment plan in this very complicated case. Also, the therapist has some work to do in terms of understanding more about the depression, if necessary by having a consultation with the physician who prescribed the medication or with her own medical consultant.

Question: I'm not sure that he had a major depression. I would ask if he had the type of depression narcissists have after they have had some kind of narcissistic injury where they have a lot of dramatic symptoms.

Dr. Tolpin: Then you explore it. Of course you're not sure about it. You have to find out about it. With the true major depression, he's got vegetative symptoms, he can't function, he can't sleep, he's lost weight or he's gained weight, his thinking becomes disorganized, and he responds to an antidepressant. That's a pretty good presumptive test that he has a depression. The answer is not clear yet to me from where we are in terms of physiological research. But I think there's a major vulnerability in terms of the biological predisposition which doesn't have a lot to do with what the psychological problems are, but enormously affects how those psychological problems are transacted.

At this time, I tend to think that there really is a strong biological element to endogenous depression. It's not set-

tled yet. That makes the person more vulnerable to everything that people are normally vulnerable to.

And I would ask you to think about one thing. You
know our diagnostic categories are so loaded with value
judgments, I don't think we should talk about the narcissist
or the borderline, etc. I understand that DSM-III-R was
an attempt to get around that. Instead of talking about the
schizophrenic, you talk about a schizophrenic disorder in
a person who has it.

I think you have to talk about the person who you feel,
if you've got to use the nomenclature, has narcissistic features. You understand that you're practicing now with that
set of nomenclature. That's going to be changed. There
will be a DSM-IV, for example. What's more, maybe the
field of psychiatry will catch on to the idea that there are
other ways of classification. For the time being, I think,
no matter what framework you use, you should try to
understand that there are a lot of built-in biases to the idea
of saying that somebody is a narcissist rather than that he
has a narcissistic disorder.

Let me tell you a classification that Kohut made about
development that's not well known. It's published in a
really wonderful article by Jewel Miller in Volume 4 of
Progress in Self Psychology, edited by Arnold Goldberg (The
Analytic Press, 1988).

Dr. Miller was the Director of the St. Louis Psychoanalytic Institute and he went to Kohut for a consultation.
He had, incidentally, worked with Erik Erikson. Somebody asked me if there were a lot of Eriksonian ideas in
Kohut. It's not so much that Kohut himself was so influenced by Erikson, but that everybody was influenced by
Erikson. It's part of an outlook that we develop towards
generativity or stagnation.

As described in this article, first of all Kohut made a
point that is very important about intervention. We do
everything we can to set up a situation in which we ask

the person to bring his problems to us and have them writ large, as it were, have them magnified—the atmosphere, the relative anonymity or neutrality, the seriousness, etc.

We set up the situation to facilitate the exposure of the problems and then, as he said to this experienced analyst, who came from the ego psychology framework and the Eriksonian work, that you then turn around and say to the patient, "But you're so sensitive to something small."

We put it under a microscope and then we say, "You're making such a big deal out of something small instead of saying it is big to you. You do experience it that way and these are the reasons that you experience it that way."

He said also that Miller's interventions often had to do with the area of greatest pathology, the greatest disintegration, and overlooked what he called the leading edge of development. So he talked about the leading edge, the intermediate area, and the trailing edge. By the leading edge, he meant those healthy aspects of the self that are in need of something. This is my association to hearing someone talk about the person with a narcissistic disorder, the person with the borderline disorder. Especially the borderline, although narcissism also has tremendous value judgments associated with it.

The health of the personality, the forward momentum that still exists, is what the leading edge is. Very often analysts were not trained to address this. Instead, they were trained to address all the areas that are in between health and the greatest disintegration and pathology, or all the pathology in the trailing edge. That is not necessarily where the fulcrum for growth and change comes from.

My point is that I think it's important to know what is part of normal development, including the idea that somebody may come to the therapist and say, "I'm in your hands." You know this is how people go to doctors. They don't expect to be an equal partner in the collaborative work with the doctor. Besides, this man has been on medication, and so forth.

So think about it in terms of what is a healthy response. It may be a healthy response to come initially and say, "Here I am." It's your job to tell the patient what's expected instead of first assuming that he's not going to do what's expected.

Now, to go on to another topic, the idea of the affective experiences is an integral part of what we're talking about.

If we say this person is "grandiose," what we mean is that there is a certain affective experience of the little kid self in this framework that was never adequately buffered and modulated and integrated and transformed into a purpose that gives life a direction. Once you have that direction, you are a much more self-sustaining, self-propelling person, which is why people lose themselves in work. They don't get sick because they work too hard, but they're sick and then they work hard trying to restore themselves, trying to give some purpose and sense of direction to their life.

The affect is in each self-configuration. The affect is in the little kid who wants to be a chip off the old block and who is putting on his father's hat and walking around or the little girl in her mother's high-heeled shoes. The affect is there of "I am a big person who is just like Mommy (or just like Daddy) and I'm bright. I'm on my way."

Whatever self-configuration exists is an affective configuration. Affect isn't separate from being enlivened. For example, Kohut talks about vitality affects. For teaching purposes, you may say they are vitality affects and there is this kind of affect and that kind of affect. What you really mean is that when that self-object unit is working and the mother looks at the child and the child looks at the mother and suddenly becomes full of energy and starts kicking and cooing and talking and carrying on an ongoing dialogue, that's a vitality affect. It's also an integral part of the whole self-configuration that is connected up, that's vitalized by being connected up, in a mutually resonating and reciprocal exhange, which is part of a normal self.

Self and object do not develop separately. This is something I've been interested in from self psychology and my interest in developmental psychology for many years. You see the self and the object developing together. It isn't that the object comes out of the self emerging from its narcissistic cocoon of splendid isolation and omnipotence.

Question: What about the abandonment depression?

Dr. Tolpin: It is inevitable that we face these experiences. Abandonment and depression, if you translate them into my framework, are all those experiences of lethargy, depletion, and deflation when you've failed to be able to elicit some life-sustaining interaction that would enable you to have the experience of being an intact self. Can you avoid that? No. You can, indeed, defend against it as much as you possibly can to preserve what you have of a self until you get into treatment where the therapist is able to tell you about your self-protective measures for holding on to the self that you have, which at the same time prevent you from being able to engage in the kind of experience that would offer you something. That's essentially another way of talking about interpretation of resistance.

Question: What is the effect on transference?

Dr. Tolpin: This also fosters transference. It also fosters alliance, as far as I'm concerned. Alliance and transference go hand in hand and much of what has been called alliance I think is a self-object transference that's operating.

I would like to briefly present a case that illustrates the split between the grandiose self and the desolate, depleted self. My patient has been in analysis for a long time. She is a talented woman therapist, gifted in many ways in working with patients. Her experience in her childhood is essentially this. She lost her father while at the same time not losing him. That is, he was there in some form and shape, but really essentially not there except occasional times that he was there in a way he was actually engaged with her. She was either his audience or there was some enlivening by their being in step with one another. They raked leaves or they rode bicycles together. There was something. He was an alternative to a mother who had fallen apart with rage and desolation at him and at the difficulties their marriage presented. My patient actually did collapse into a major depression during her adolescence, for which she had to be hospitalized. She made a recovery, but she still had a thought disorder and became almost totally self absorbed. But she never had a complete breakdown.

So the patient is one of these talented people, a lot of drive, a professional person working at a fairly high level who, in essence, felt that she was a fraud. That she had had it, that everybody responded to her as, "Oh you, you know you're this and you're that and you've got this and you do this." Within herself, she was depressed, she was flat, she could be a cheerleader type with other people but within herself she was depressed and flat and she felt fraudulent.

In the stage of the analysis that I'll tell you about to illustrate these configurations, she had a surge of interest in doing something that she was asked to do—to give a lecture. She asked a friend, also in the field, to participate with her in doing this. Then she began to suffer from her feeling that she was a fraud and that the friend was the only one who had it.

So I asked her to tell me more about how this happned to her, with the surge of enthusiasm and then the old experience of feeling so fraudulent. She said, "At first when I talked to my friend about it, I thought we were going to be like Siskel and Ebert, reviewing films together. We were really going to enter into this dialogue and it will be challenging and interesting and stimulating for the audience." That feeling lasted about 15 minutes and then it collapsed. I said, "What does it collapse into?" And she said suddenly, and this was a really spontaneous free association, that she didn't usually talk about this, but it was into a lost little girl.

And then she told me again about material that had been part of the analysis but not in this context of the collapse of her great expectations about herself, the Siskel and Ebert feeling that we're going to be great.

I asked, "What about that?" And she said, "You know about that." And then she told me about all the times she had gone to the bus station hoping that her father would be there and he never was. Then she would have a dream the next day. The dream was about the defensive isolation of this experience of being the lost little girl on the one hand and part of a magnificent pair on the other. It is still part of this self-configuration.

Then she came back with this dream. She is lying on the couch in my office, during analysis and she is looking out of the window and she sees the Magnificent Mile—a part of North Lakeshore Drive in Chicago, with fancy stores and buildings. Suddenly it crumbles, it just disintegrates.

Although patients learn to talk your theory once you've got your theory together, still it's in the background and you don't talk to the patients in theoretical language, such as the disintegration of a grandiose self. She says the Magnificent Mile just crumbles and she is terror-struck, in a total panic, and she turns to me in the dream for recognition, validation that she's seeing what she's seeing. But I either don't see it or I'm trying to minimize it so I don't acknowledge that I've seen it and that makes her even more terrified because then she thinks she's going crazy. Did she see it or didn't she see it?

What I tell her, in essence, is that she had this surge of excitement, but people take a very pejorative attitude towards their own narcissism. Patients have the attitude that the therapist has made this classification of narcissism. So the patient says "I'm grandiose, there is my grandiosity again," or "There is my narcissism," because she is ashamed of it and has to defend. So she defends herself against it by saying, "I know about that, I know I'm a narcissist."

So I said that she was still struggling with this issue where she got excited and had these great expectations of herself, that she was terrified that she would not be able to be that great self because she always had felt depleted and flat and isolated. On the one hand she's the great self and on the other hand she's the lost little girl. These two have been apart, that's the vertical split. I don't like that term either, but it was meant to convey that the feeling is in the conscious mind. There are side by side configurations that are separated by a wall of defense, but it's not like repression. The treatment is explanation and understanding of the configurations. The things that would make her believe in herself were, indeed, very deficient.

This is a little girl who went over and over and over again hoping to find the father, to separate herself from the mother who was falling apart and raging against the father who wasn't there. Or even if he was there, he never came to school, neither parent ever came to school, neither parent ever saw her perform. Her father never knew the names of any of her friends. Her mother did know the names of her friends. She turned to alternatives, alter egos, girls that she was friendly with whose mothers responded to her and took her in and even bought her clothes. But she felt like a lost little girl, a beggar, an orphan. The very things that made people respond to her made her also feel like she was a beggar and a fraud.

This is what we talked about. I told her that I would minimize the feeling of going crazy, that I would not validate that she was in any danger of collapsing evey time she had a surge of feeling great. The development since that time has been that she got into a spurt of work where she wrote out her talk and where she used a book she had read on the subject, which she previously had been afraid to use because she thought she would be fraudulent, just a plagiarist. Nobody without this kind of disorder would feel he was robbing somebody by using material in the public domain. But for grandiose expectations, you have to do it all yourself or else you're taking away from somebody else, or you're taking it away from this desperately ill mother, and so on.

What is the process that goes on? The process is the explanation, which Masterson talked about as communicative matching. This patient now knows she has to work at something in order to sustain the grandiose expectation. She couldn't do it without the validation that I understood what the problem was—that she collapses every time she sets up because she cannot sustain it within herself.

There was a little bit more, a firmness in her resolution and less fear of being a fraud and not being able to undertake the work.

12

Final Discussion

Question: I have two questions about the idealizing transference. First, to what extent is the idealized transference really in the work and truly allowed to spontaneously come into being, as long as we don't prevent it from doing so? Or is there a more active attempt on the part of the therapist to bring about the idealizing transference?

As a follow-up to that question about the idealizing transference, how does one understand the interventions associated with managing the transference in terms of therapeutic neutrality? What different interventions are necessary in order to manage the idealizing transference for the purpose of therapeutic change and growth?

Dr. Tolpin: Do you foster an idealizing transference or do you permit its "spontaneous enfolding," or, and this is the third possibility, do you not interfere with it? No you do not foster it. Freud said in a footnote that the analyst cannot play prophet, savior, or redeemer. I think that is basic orientation for therapists. You have a whole attitude towards a patient that comes out of your overall training and your total commitment as a therapist.

Physicians are automatically magnets for transference. This process is what you bring to it. It is you and your training and your therapeutic attitude and commitment that make you into an idealizable person. In order to develop, children need to have idealizable, mirroring alter ego functions available for them from the people whom they contact. However, you don't need to do anything but be what you are, with the therapeutic equipment, skills, knowledge, methods you bring to the therapy.

Will it unfold spontaneously? Possibly. Probably the type of transference the patient develops is uniquely characteristic of that individual. Will it be affected by who and what you are? Very likely. All this could be studied in detail and then we could say more about it, but some people, especially when they're starting out in therapy, are magnets for what Kohut called twinship or alter ego transferences.

I used to think the patient was dreaming about me as though I were her girlfriend. This was long before there was a description of what I could, even in the present era, call loosely a girlfriend transference. A young therapist I know was a magnet for that kind of transference and patients whom she had treated often would make referrals to her because they had experienced something like that. It becomes a unique amalgam of what you are, your style, and what you have learned.

Not interfering with it is a crucial part of the question because many theories interfere with it. The theory that it is invariably a defensive move against hostility, for example, is an interference. If you have that theory and you operate with it, bite your tongue or keep your mouth closed and see what happens. Of course, it will permeate the atmosphere if you really feel negatively about it, about the patient, or about your countertransference. You think,

"Who, me? I'm not so ideal. I'm not so idealizable." You have to debunk it that way.

In our workshop, a young woman therapist said the patient was too passive and didn't act as if he was participating. Then she proceeded to give this wonderful account of all the things he had told her about himself and his inner world.

Thus, whether she knew it or not, he had come to her with the anticipation of finding somebody he could unburden himself to with expectations that she was going to understand. That's the kind of precursor of a remobilization of a normal experience in childhood in which we ran to our parents and said, "Kiss it and make it well."

The answer is yes and no. It will spontaneously unfold if you don't interfere with it. The answer is a decided no to fostering it.

Dr. Sifneos: I would like to direct a question both to Dr. Tolpin and to Dr. Masterson. In the third interview a patient comes in, maybe after an evaluation where some things were stirred up, and says, "Dr. Tolpin, I notice today you're wearing a beautiful new scarf." And that's that. "Dr. Masterson, I like your blue tie." Do you leave it? Do you pick it up? Do you proceed to get more information? I was wondering how you would handle such a situation?

Dr. Tolpin: It gets into the question of what therapeutic neutrality is.

The first thing I do now is say, "Thank you," and I tuck it away. I think about it. I wonder about it. I think about its meanings and it goes into the whole experience. Do I immediately decide the patient is seducing me, buttering me up, trying to manipulate me? I don't decide about any of those things . . . It is part of the data.

In addition, although I don't think any of us are such perfect instruments in reading people right the first time around, I may have some vibes because of the affective part of it; I may cringe a little because the patient is in-gratiating. There are all sorts of nonverbal cues that are going to evoke something in me. But I don't do anything at that point except to politely say, "Thank you." And this response is part of my idea of therapeutic neutrality these days.

Dr. Masterson: Being a real person, you mean.

Dr. Tolpin: There is no question that therapists are real persons. There never has been. So it is permitted to know that you are and to show that.

Dr. Masterson: Let's take it a step further. Suppose this patient develops a pattern of starting off the interview with a com-ment about you as opposed to herself? What happens then?

Dr. Tolpin: Then you begin to read it in terms of whether or not it is a displacement. Is it an avoidance or a retreat? Assuming that is one of these things, I might say, "Thank you very much. I notice that you are very involved with or attentive to the things that I wear." I would first of all make it as broad an umbrella or net as possible so I don't immediately prejudice it with some kind of premature closure as to what it means. Actually, the patient now will immediately feel criticized, no matter what, no matter how, so I will be aware of that.

Dr. Masterson: I would not agree with your last statement. I think it depends on the kind of patient. Without question, a narcissistic patient would feel criticized. Let me give you an example of before I learned something more about these matters.

Some years ago when I began to do treatment, I had this patient who was a top salesman. He had a borderline personality disorder, upper level, with a lot of clinging defenses. He also was on the Board of Trustees at Cornell

New York Hospital and no sooner had we started treatment than I learned from him that at every board meeting of the Hospital my name was prominently mentioned and everyone thought I was a terrific psychiatrist. I recognized that he was trying to seduce me. However, instead of identifying it for what it was and reflecting it, I reacted to it by getting angry. I knew enough even then not to tell him my anger. As a result, my emotional flexibility froze in the sessions. I was more concerned about my anger than about what he was saying. Then, he switched from this kind of seduction to attacking me for being a cold fish. And he was right, I was. I also was in analysis at the time and I finally got to work out what was going on inside.

Then I came back to ask him why he felt the need to seduce me into being interested in him.

How would I handle it now with a borderline patient in the third interview? If I had a consistent picture from the evaluation interview that his principal mechanism of defense was clinging, and if we had talked about something in a second interview that was disturbing, and if I'm seeing him twice a week so there is enough possibility of continuity, I probably would not say thank you. I might say, "I am struck by the fact that as you came in here your first reaction was to focus on me rather than on yourself." These comments have to be dealt with in context. I agree with you that if I were ambivalent about it, if I weren't sure, I'd keep my mouth shut until I had figured it out. Once the patient is in treatment, I think you have the time. In other words, if you can't figure out what you want to do, if you don't have confidence in it, keep your mouth shut and don't do anything. You can't get in trouble for what you didn't say. So I would wait until I had figured it out and then I would do something.

If a similar situation arose with a narcissistic disorder, I would explore it with him. I might say, "I wonder why your first reaction was to talk about me? What occurs to you about that? How does this compare with other situations?" I try to explore it with him a bit.

If the treatment were far enough along, I might do the narcissistic vulnerability interpretation as opposed to the confrontation. "I suspect it's painful for you to focus on yourself here and one way to soothe the pain is to talk about me, the way I look, the way I behave, and so forth."

Dr. Sifneos: It's very interesting, really, because this shows what I think is the essence of what this conference is all about and the differences in terms of the kinds of patients we are dealing with. Dr. Tolpin's approach is, of course, very cautious about this, not to get involved in the kinds of patients that she would see. Dr. Masterson says he might inquire with some and with others he would let it go.

Let me tell you about what happened, for instance, with one of the patients we had in short-term therapy. "I notice that you're wearing a new tie today." "Please tell me what are your thoughts about my new tie." "Oh, come on, I was just making small talk." "No, I'm very much interested in your thoughts about my new tie." After a silence, he said, "Come to think of it, it reminds me of something." "Yes, tell me more about what it reminds you of." "Well, my older brother used to have a tie that looked a bit like yours." "Oh, what about your older brother?" "Well, I had problems, as you know, with my father and my mother and they always criticized me. He always took my side. He always protected me and he always essentially was tying to defend me against them and so forth." "So you mean you were quite close to your older brother?" "Oh, yes, very much so."

There we have a past/present link between things that have existed. And the patient is saying he wants you to protect him and he likes you because of whatever it is, which to us is very valuable and can be utilized early in the therapy.

Dr. Masterson: You're doing it again. You're driving me crazy because it's so comparatively easy for you to get to the heart of the problem. Why is Dr. Tolpin so cautious and why am I so cautious? From my point of view, we don't have the therapeutic alliance you have. That is our principal concern and that is what severely limits our operation. Without that, we can't get from the past to the present. The key to getting the past link with the present is therapeutic alliance. You start out with it. We struggle in the trenches for months to get to the point where we have achieved a therapeutic alliance and the emotional stage is set to link past with present.

In classical analytic treatment, you can do things like that because you know that you have the therapeutic alliance and it's sound.

I know that some people view idealizing as a defense against rage. My view is that it is defensive, not against rage but against the fragmented self. And so I consider it defensive but allow it, knowing that if I don't interfere with it, it is going to reveal itself in the transference acting out.

Dr. Tolpin: The trouble with theory and with the way people learn a theory is it doesn't give you a range of options. One of the things that Kohut said was that one should think not obsessionally but reviewing as many possibilities as one can before coming to a closure.

First of all, Dr. Sifneos' response belongs to a whole theoretical outlook that considers that the past is transferred onto the present onto the person of the analyst. Thus, he has sieved this communication through that framework. Second, he hears it as facilitating or positive for what he's trying to do. He's trying to see the potential for establishing a quick transference-like bond and then using it purposefully.

He's not doing an exploration of whether or not this is

beginning alter ego transference that he's identified with the brother whom she could turn to as an alternative who was helpful. He is not asking, "Is it the beginning of this or that?" No. In his framework and the type of research he has committed himself to he has to make rapid clinical judgments. He builds on them and he trusts his hunch as a seasoned clinician. Somebody else can raise questions about it, but this is how he has decided he's going to proceed.

You cannot compare his method and how he hears it with the way you and I hear it. He has a different objective.

Dr. Masterson: We can compare the differences in clinical material and method of approach. It's true that he has a different objective and method. He also has the type of patient who presents different phenomena than the kinds of phenomena presented to us. Therefore, he deals with them in a different way. But it is this difference that uniquely highlights and helps to explain the phenomena we deal with.

Dr. Tolpin: He doesn't have the follow-up now, so we don't know whose couch that young lady ends up on.

Dr. Sifneos: No, I wouldn't say that. I have very intensive follow-up. Not only that, but we have done exactly the same work in Norway. We don't have five or seven years as they have in Norway. They have 90% follow-up which they have written about statistically. But let me just point out one thing about this past/present link interpretation. David Malin at the Tavistock Clinic was able to assess criterion one, motivation for change, a crucial criterion for selection. From excellent notes he could statistically predict change from the number of past-present interpretations done in the first five interviews.

Dr. Masterson: Just the number of interpretations, and not whether they're timed properly or phrased properly?

Dr. Sifneos: Right. Obviously they assumed they are. This raises an issue that Jerome Frank talked about, the essence of psychotherapy being the so-called non-specific factors of support and various other things. Here are two things. A criterion for selection and a technical device that is being used for this type of patient that produces a successful outcome on sophisticated criteria. No! My patients don't end on anybody's couch. Thank goodness for that.

Dr. Masterson: Dr. Tolpin, what's being done in the field of self psychology about follow-ups?

Dr. Tolpin: Whether there's systematic study right now, I can't tell you. It's like any other development in psychoanalysis and applied psychoanalysis, meaning psychotherapy. There is a lot of clinical work being done and there isn't any systematic follow-up, except that all of us have follow-ups.

Our patients either come back to us or go to somebody else. In that sense we have follow-up. One of the important things, in my view, is that psychoanalytic theory originally sold itself a bill of goods on the notion of what change consists of.

This young woman overcame a developmental road-block at that time. Dr. Sifneos thought she was on the right track. In the three and one-half year follow-up, he found out that she was no longer in relationships where she felt she was either controlled or controlling. She was 27 at the time of the follow-up.

She had overcome a developmental issue that was interfering with her adult growth. What was her adult growth? One would want to know for an adequate follow-up. Do you have to do everything? No. Surely he doesn't have to do everything in an eight-session design which is attempting to deal with the focal problem in a focal way. Should very long-term treatment four times a week do everything? The answer is yes, of course, ideally it should.

It turns out that it doesn't. It turns out, in terms of what
the self psychological outlook would be, it does marvelously for some people just as a therapeutic encounter of
brief duration does marvelously for some people. There
is a whole spectrum of results.

What's more, we are changing the whole notion of cure
and what we're trying to accomplish. If you can overcome
a developmental impediment that is interfering with the
next stage of development, wonderful. You do it in eight
interviews if you can. You do it in a year's treatment if
you can. You do it twice a week if you can.

If you cannot do that, if development really is significantly offtrack, you may then think that you can do it in
much more intensive and prolonged work. And all of these
things have to be investigated in complicated, methodological ways that are in their infancy. But there is no reason
not to think that maybe what you do in all treatments is
shift the balance. And if you shift that balance, it's enough
for some people to be able to go forward in their momentum instead of always falling back. Thus, if you have
a criterion like that, you may have a wide range of possibilities that are opened up to you in terms of deciding
what kind of therapy it should be.

Would you accept that, Dr. Sifneos, as your definition
of cure?

Dr. Sifneos: I accept it completely, but I want to ask one more
question addressed to both of you again. One of the findings in our follow-ups, some after five years, some after
three years, is the statement of the patient having faced a
new emotional problem in his life. Patients say, "I am
thinking the kinds of questions that my therapist would
have asked me if I were in therapy. I ask these questions
in my own head. And I answer it back and forth. That
helps me solve the problem in the same way as I learned

to solve problems in my therapy." I call that internalized dialogue.

One amusing example is a patient of mine, a lady whom I saw five years later. She told me just that. She said, "I had this problem, Dr. Sifneos, and I was thinking of the kinds of questions you would have asked me back and forth, and so forth, and it didn't work out. Then I imitated your accent and it did work out." I felt narcissistically very pleased by that. Really, what this lady was saying was that she was carrying this thing that she had learned from the therapy in her own head and therefore she was independent of me, of anybody else. Isn't that what we do also in our own analysis? Can't we really remember the kinds of questions that our own analysts used to ask about us?

Dr. Tolpin: Kohut had a very interesting idea about the so-called self-analytic function that people are supposed to develop in analysis, especially if they are going to be in the field. But you're talking about a kind of approach, a life approach, that somebody in short-term work can carry away.

Kohut said that he wouldn't call it self-analytic, but rather a problem-solving approach. He said that maybe the self-analytic function everybody talks about in analytic theory is really an emergency measure. You call in the image and the voice and the experience with the analyst when you are in some emergency state where the imbalance is such that the self-righting capacities aren't working and so you fill this in with a reevocation of the actual person of the analyst. Even in a short-term therapy, what a powerful influence it is to have available to you this kind of helping hand when you're in the quicksand. How meaningful it is and how it resonates in your whole development to have somebody available to you for that, for you carry it with you forever.

Dr. Masterson: Let me comment first on the follow-up issue. For example, as far as your self psychology group is concerned, I guess from one perspective in the development of science you might say it's too early or perhaps a very early stage for follow-up study, that you're really putting down your parameters in a solid way and want to do that before you follow up.

I am a veteran of follow-up studies. I have done three follow-up studies in my lifetime. These consumed some 30 years of toil and trouble and I found out why people don't do follow-up studies: They don't want to find out what actually happens because it interferes with all their fantasies about what happens.

I did a follow-up study on the treatment of borderline adolescents. We had marvelous clinical methodological data. These patients were hospitalized for 14 months and we had the whole treatment record. Then we followed them up seven years later. I reported results in a book *From Borderline Adolescent to Functioning Adult: The Test of Time* (Brunner/Mazel, 1980). The results were analogous to what you were saying. We sketched out a sequence from the testing phase through the working-through phase to the separation phase. And we described the clinical parameters of each of those phases. We were able to make a highly statistically significant prediction of outcome by reviewing the hospital record to determine the degree to which they went through these phases as they were supposed to.

I think even in the personality disorders follow-up studies are only beginning. In our follow-up studies, we interviewed every adolescent and every set of parents. I don't have a lot of faith in follow-up studies that are done by telephone or mail.

Finally, I was having a kind of déjà-vu as Dr. Sifneos was talking, because I had had a similar experience. It's as if these two patients were talking to each other. This was a young woman with a borderline disorder who tended to relate to men who would devalue her. Some years after treatment, she prematurely got together with a man and she took off with him on a trip to India. When she got to India, he started to attack her. Borderline patients' lack of object constancy provides enough difficulties in their own country, but in a foreign country where there's no structural support, they can regress. The more he attacked her, the more she regressed and clung to him. Then she reported, "One night I was lying in bed and it was as if I could hear your voice saying, 'Why are you letting him do this to you? Why aren't you doing something about yourself?' So I did and he didn't go along with it, so I left him."

Thus, I think it very much does happen.

Dr. Tolpin: There is a lot of clinical judgment that can tell you what some of the findings are before doing these careful follow-up studies. I don't mean to be provocative or "unscientific," but in a clinical analytic practice, you can say that a third of the people get dramatically better, a third get somewhat better or stay the same, and a third stay the same.

Those were the original figures of Pinel who studied what happened to people in institutions for the insane in Paris.

I think that honest clinicians will tell you it is not a scientific field. It is an art where you hope your art is schooled in some basic psychological understanding of human beings and how to affect them. But why do you think there are all these theories? Why do you think we're having conferences like this? Why do clinicians want to hear about self psychology and why do they flock to the self psychology conferences and why are they looking forward to the next innovation in psychoanalytic theory? It's because results aren't good enough, because we're looking to improve the results.

I think the development of self psychology is enormously important because there used to be a kind of élitism in psychoanalysis and a lot of misunderstandings connected with the élitism. One was that treatment was good only if you went four times a week for four or five years. That was the only way of working through problems.

We know that that's not so now. We know that you shift the balance for some people and they go on from there. We have learned more. But we still haven't learned enough. At each stage of clinical therapy we're beset with problems that we don't do well enough with. That is why we go to conferences like this one.

PART III

Overview

13

Comparing Psychoanalytic Psychotherapies

James F. Masterson, M.D.

Theory is a powerful agent to help the therapist refine his observations and interventions, but only so long as its limitations are kept in mind. The theory must be subordinated to the clinical data rather than the data being compressed to fit the theory. The theory must not blind the therapist to observations of clinical data that do not fit. In other words, it is a tool, not a master.

The cases presented in this volume served as excellent vehicles to allow the three experts to demonstrate how their theory influences what they observe, how they organize these observations to make a diagnosis, and how that diagnosis determines when and how they intervene and the responses they anticipate from those interventions. A number of systematic themes of difference emerged from the case discussions and workshops. The differences between Dr. Sifneos and the other two experts were due to the fact that the type of patient he focused on had an essentially different disorder, that is, a neurosis rather than a personality disorder. The differences between Dr. Masterson and Dr. Tolpin were due to differing theoretical approaches to the personality disorder. I shall try to summarize these differences under the following headings:

- Assumption as to Basic Pathology and its Etiology
- Diagnosis
- Approach to Psychotherapy
- Assumption of the Effective Agent in Psychotherapy

The reader should keep in mind that the views of each of the therapists have been condensed to provide an essential contrast. What is lost in complexity may be gained by the contrast. For a fuller view, the reader should consult each author's publications (see Bibliography).

MASTERSON

Assumption as to Basic Pathology and its Etiology

The basic pathology of the borderline and narcissistic personality disorders is a developmental arrest or impairment of the self due to one or all of three factors: (1) genetic defects; (2) separation stress; and (3) the mother's difficulties in supporting the individuative, emerging aspect of the self. The final common clinical pathway is that real self-activation leads to separation anxiety and to abandonment depression, that leads to defense. The patient has the capacity for self-activation, but the need to defend against the depression keeps it from being activated. The therapeutic intervention removing these defenses enables the patient to work through the depression and overcome the developmental arrest.

Diagnosis

Symptoms are a reflection of the defenses against the abandonment depression that is associated with self-activation. The symptoms as described in DSM-III are used as initial clinical evidence, but the basic diagnosis is made on the basis of intrapsychic structure, that is, self and object representations and ego functions and defense mechanisms. The borderline personality disorder has a different intrapsychic structure than the narcissistic personality disorder and requires a different therapeutic approach. Therefore, it is important to make a differential diagnosis between these two types of disorders.

Approach to Psychotherapy

The objective of the psychotherapy is to help the patient convert his/her transference acting-out to therapeutic alliance and transference. This is done in the borderline personality disorder by confrontation and in the narcissistic personality disorder through mirroring interpretations of narcisstic vulnerability. These interventions enable the patient to overcome his/her defenses against the rage and depression of the abandonment depression associated with self-activation and to work through these pathologic affects, thus freeing the emerging self from that burden and allowing it to overcome the developmental arrest and grow and take on its functions.

Assumption of the Effective Agent in Psychotherapy

The establishment of the therapeutic alliance in reality where the patient's self-activation is supported serves as a background against which the fantasies of transference can be identified, measured, and worked through. It is the contrast between the two which provides the essential framework for the patient to work through his anger and depression associated with his/her transference projections. It is the frustration inherent in the contrast between transference fantasy and the reality of therapeutic alliance that promotes internalization of therapeutic interventions and repair of the self.

SIFNEOS

Assumption as to Basic Pathology and its Etiology

The patient suffers from a neurotic disorder, such as a conflict between the id and the super ego which is beyond the awareness of the ego. In contrast to the personality disorders, the patient has a fully activated, consolidated self able to perform all its functions.

Diagnosis

Diagnosis is made on the basis of the following six criteria: (1) *Acute onset* of a (2) *circumscribed symptom* in a patient in (3) *crisis* who is (4) *psychologically minded*, has had a (5) *good relationship* with at least one person in childhood, and has demonstrated a (6) *good interpersonal interaction* with the therapist on initial evaluation. These last three characteristics help to differentiate the neurotic from the personality disorders. They reflect the fact that the patient has an effective consolidated self. This gives the therapist much greater leeway for therapeutic intervention.

Approach to Psychotherapy

The psychotherapy focuses on rapid, active mobilization of the already existing therapeutic alliance and genetic interpretations contrasting the past with the present, bringing to the awareness of the patient's ego the conflicting forces that underlie the symptom. These interpretations are, however, limited to the forces that underly the focal conflict reflected in the symptoms. Other aspects are not focused on.

Assumption of the Effective Agent in Psychotherapy

The contrast between the therapeutic alliance and the transference allows the patient, when his/her transference projections are interpreted, to become aware of the conflict, which then allows the ego to redistribute the forces that had produced a neurotic symptom.

TOLPIN

Assumption as to Basic Pathology and its Etiology

The basic pathology of the Disorders of the Self (both borderline personality disorder and narcissistic personality disorder) is viewed as a defect in the structure of the self due to failure of the self-object functions of the parents. The assumption, in contrast to the Masterson Approach, is that the patient does not have the capacity for self-activation and requires the self-functions of the therapist in order to internalize them and activate the self.

Diagnosis

There are dramatic differences from the Masterson Approach to diagnosis. DSM-III symptoms are not utilized and emphasis is placed strictly on the observable defects in the structure of the self and on the form of self-object transference, that is, the way the patient relates to the therapist. Symptoms are seen not as defensive but as the result of efforts to compensate for or repair the defect in the self.

There is no recognition of the existence of a separate diagnostic category for the borderline as a personality disorder, only as a borderline psychotic. Otherwise, the borderline personality disorder is viewed as just another form of narcissistic disorder. Differential diagnosis, then, is not between one kind of disorder and another, but between different degrees of the same disorder. In other words, they are both disorders of the self which differ only in degree.

Approach to Psychotherapy

The psychotherapy consists of the management through interpretation of the self-object transference. This concept of transference differs from the usual notion. It is defined as that part of the patient's fragmented self that turns to the therapist for the self-object functions that were not available in childhood. The therapist's empathic understanding and interpretations supply the missing self-object functions, which are internalized by the patient, allowing the self to overcome its trauma, grow, and assume its functions. Inevitable disruptions and disappointments in this self-object transference search occur which are then interpreted. This view stresses that what matters is not reality, but the patient's feelings and perceptions, as well as the fact that the focus through the agency of empathy must be on the patient's feelings and perceptions.

Assumption of the Effective Agent in Psychotherapy

The patient experiences the therapist's encouragement of self-activation and understanding and interpretations of the disruptions of self-object transference as providing those missing self-object functions that the parents failed to provide. Through transmuting internalizations, he/she uses them to repair his/her fragmented self.

DISCUSSION

In the Sifneos approach to the neuroses, it is clear that the consolidated self of the patient allows the therapist to act more quickly, to go deeper, and to get a stronger response. In other words, the therapist can offer interpretations in early sessions, while work with personality disorders requires many months of groundwork in order to prepare the patient to be ready to utilize such interventions.

There are vast differences between Masterson's and Tolpin's views on the borderline and narcissistic personality disorders. These differences cover a wide range, from the assumption of what is wrong through how one goes about making the diagnosis, as well as the assumptions regarding the kinds of treatment offered and what is the effective agent of treatment. Masterson viewed the basic pathology as an arrest of the self, which nevertheless had capacity for self-activation that has been held in check by the need to defend against abandonment depression. Alleviating the depression allows the self to become active. Tolpin stresses that the basic pathology is a defect in the structure of the self due to failure of parents' self-object functions and the patient does not have the capacity for self-activation. S/he develops this capacity through internalizing the therapist's self-object functions.

Their views of diagnosis also differ. Masterson used symptomatology only initially and bases diagnosis on the intrapsychic structure. Beyond that, he stresses the importance of differentiating between the borderline personality disorder and the narcissistic personality disorder. He views them as two different kinds of personality disorders that require different therapeutic interventions.

Tolpin bases diagnosis on the defects in the structure of the self and on the type of self-object transference. She sees no difference in the disorders of the self between the borderline personality disorder and the narcissistic personality disorders. The difference is seen as one only of degree, not of kind, so that the borderline personality disorder receives the same treatment as the narcissistic disorder. (The borderline psychotic seems different.)

These differences, as might be expected, are also carried out in their views of psychotherapy. Masterson stresses that the task is to undo the defenses, establish a therapeutic alliance, encourage self-activation, and help the patient convert his/her transference acting-out into therapeutic alliance and transference. It is this very conversion which sets the reality framework of the therapeutic alliance that is essential as a contrast to the transference projections. These are then used to work through the rage and depression associated with self-activation, freeing the self from the pathologic affects and allowing it to grow and take on its functions.

Tolpin, on the other hand, stresses the management of the self-object transference through encouragement of self-activation, as well as through interpretations of disruptions in the self-object transference. These activities provide the missing self-object functions which the patient internalizes in order to promote the growth of the self. This approach minimizes the therapeutic alliance and reality, stressing instead the use of empathic understanding of the patient's feeling states. In addition, since the borderline personality disorder is not differentiated from the narcissistic personality disorder, both receive the same treatment.

In my clinical experience, attempting to use narcissistic mirroring interpretations with borderline patients has always led to regression and a therapeutic stalemate, since the therapist is reinforcing the patient's rewarding-unit projections. The patient feels good, but the momentum of treatment stops.

I also have serious questions as to whether or not Dr. Tolpin's emphasis on empathy and the patient's feeling states, while minimizing reality and the therapeutic alliance, reinforces the patient's transference acting-out of his narcissistic projection in such a manner that the force of therapeutic interpretation is diluted. There is no countervailing therapeutic alliance to serve as a framework of contrast.

It is axiomatic in this field that the fact that the patient gets better is in no way proof of the theory. Ostensibly the patients of all three experts get better or we wouldn't be in this discussion. We have tried in this volume to clarify these differences in such a way that the reader can come to his or her own decisions.

Bibliography

by James F. Masterson

1972 *Treatment of the borderline adolescent: A developmental approach.* New York: Wiley.

1973 The tie that binds: Maternal clinging, separation-individuation and the borderline syndrome. *Internatinoal Journal of Child Psychotherapy, 2,* 331–344.

1975 With Rinsley, D. B. The borderline syndrome: The role of the mother in the genesis and psychic structure of the borderline personality. *International Journal of Psychoanalysis, 56.*

1976 *Psychotherapy of the borderline adult: A dedvelopmental approach.* New York: Brunnel/Mazel.

1978 Therapeutic alliance and transference. *American Journal of Psychiatry, 135*(4), 435–441.

1978 The borderline adult: Transference acting out and working through. *New perspectives on psychotherapy of the borderline adult* (Chap. 4). New York: Brunner/Mazel.

1981 *Narcissistic and borderline disorders: An integrated developmental approach.* New York: Brunner/Mazel.

1983 *Countertransference and psychotherapeutic technique: Teaching seminars on psychotherapy of the borderline adult.* New York: Brunner/Mazel.

1985 *The real self: A developmental, self and object relations approach.* New York: Brunner/Mazel.

1988 *The search for the real self: Unmasking the personality disorders of our age.* New York: Free Press.

1988 With Klein, R. (Eds.). *Psychotherapy of the disorders of the self: The Masterson approach.* New York: Brunner/Mazel.

by Marian Tolpin

1970 The infantile neurosis. *Psychoanalytic Study of the Child, 25,* 273–305.

1971 On the beginnings of a cohesive self. *Psychoanalytic Study of the Child, 26,* 316–352.

1974 The Daedulus experience. *Annual of Psychoanalysis, 2,* 213–228.

1978 Self-objects and oedipal objects: A crucial developmental distinction. *Psychoanalytic Study of the Child, 33,* 167–186.

1978 *The psychology of the self: A casebook.* (Contributing Eds.: Goldberg, A., Basch, M. F., Gunther, M. S., Marcus, D., Ornstein, A., Ornstein, P., Tolpin, M., Tolpin, P., Wolf, E.) New York: International Universities Press.

1978 Discussion of Levine, H. B., Sustaining object relationship. *Annual of Psychoanalysis, 7,* 219–225.

1980 With Kohut, H. The disorders of the self—The psychopathology of the first years of life. In S. Greenspan & G. Pollock, (Eds.), *The course of life* (Vol. I, pp. 425–442). Washington, DC: U.S. Government Printing Office.

1980 Discussion of Shane, M., & Shane, E., Psychoanalytic theories of the self: An integration. In A. Goldberg (Ed.), *Advances in self psychology.* New York: International Universities Press.

1982 Book review: Little, M., *Transference neurosis, transference psychosis.* Journal of the American Psychiatric Association.

1983 Corrective emotional experience: A self psychological re-evaluation. In A. Goldberg (Ed.), *The future of psychoanalysis.* New York: International Universities Press.

1983 Discussion of papers by Drs. Stern and Sander. In J. Lichtenberg & S. Kaplan (Eds.), *Reflections on self psychology* (pp. 113–123). Hillsdale, NJ: Analytic Press.

1986 The self and its selfobjects—A different baby. In A. Goldberg (Ed.), *Progress in self psychology,* (Vol. II). New York: International Universities Press.

1987 Toward the metapsychology of injured self-cohesion. In J. Grotstein, J. Lang, & M. Solomon (Eds.), *The borderline patient.* Hillsdale, NJ: Analytic Press.

1987 Discussion of Black, M. J., The analyst's stance: Transferential implications of technical orientation. *Annual of Psychoanalysis,* *15*, 159–164.

1989 Discussion of Demos, V., A prospective constructionist view of development. *Annual Review of Psychoanalysis.*

by Peter E. Sifneos

1964 *Ascent from chaos. A psychosomatic case study.* Cambridge, MA: Harvard University Press.

1966 Motivation for psychotherapy of short duration. In *Proceedings of the Fourth World Congress of Psychiatry,* Madrid, Spain. (Also *Excerpta Medica,* 1968, Part III.)

1968 Learning to solve emotional problems: A controlled study of short-term psychotherapy. In *The Role of Learning in Psychotherapy* (pp. 87–96). London: J. & A. Churchill.

1972 *Short-term dynamic psychotherapy evaluation and technique.* New York: Plenum.

1972/73 Is dynamic psychotherapy contraindicated for a large number of patients with psychosomatic disorders? *Psychotherapy and Psychosomatics, 27,* 133–136.

1978 Short-term anxiety provoking psychotherapy. In H. Davanloo (Ed.), *Short-term dynamic psychotherapy* (pp. 35–42). New York: Spectrum.

1978 Evaluation criteria for selection of patients. In H. Davanloo (Ed.), *Short-term dynamic psychotherapy* (pp. 81–85). New York: Spectrum.

1978 The case of the Italian housewife. In H. Davanloo (Ed.), *Short-term dynamic psychotherapy* (pp. 99–129). New York: Spectrum.

1978 The case of the college student. In H. Davanloo (Ed.), *Short-term dynamic psychotherapy* (pp. 159–171). New York: Spectrum.

1979 *Short-term dynamic psychotherapy evaluation and technique.* New York: Plenum.

1980 Brief psychotherapy and crisis intervention. In Kaplan, H., Freedman, A. M., & Saddock, B. D. (Eds.), *Comprehensive textbook of psychiatry* (3rd ed., Vol. II, pp. 2247–2257). New York: Williams & Wilkins.

1983 With Nemiah, J. C. Assessing the suitability of patients with character disorders for insight psychotherapy. In M. R. Zales (Ed.), *Character pathology* (pp. 119–130). New York: Brunner/ Mazel.

1984 The current status of short-term dynamic psychotherapy and its future. *American Journal of Psychotherapy, 38*(4).

For Product Safety Concerns and Information please contact our
EU representative GPSR@taylorandfrancis.com Taylor & Francis
Verlag GmbH, Kaufingerstraße 24, 80331 München, Germany